NUTRITION IN
HEALTH AND DISEASE

NUTRITION IN HEALTH AND DISEASE

MYRON WINICK, M.D.

Institute of Human Nutrition Columbia University
College of Physicians and Surgeons

A WILEY-INTERSCIENCE PUBLICATION

JOHN WILEY & SONS, New York • Chichester • Brisbane • Toronto

Library of Congress Cataloging in Publication Data:

Winick, Myron.
  Nutrition in health and disease.

  "A Wiley-Interscience publication."
  Includes index.
  1. Nutrition. 2. Diet in disease. I. Title.
[DNLM: 1. Nutrition disorders. 2. Nutrition.
3. Diet therapy. WD100 W772n]

QP141.W533   613.2   80-13566
ISBN 0-471-05713-4

Printed in the United States of America

10 9 8 7 6 5 4 3 2 1

PREFACE

Many medical schools have set up or are in the process of setting up courses in nutrition for undergraduate medical students. In addition, many graduate physicians, both in and out of training, have expressed the desire to obtain more fundamental knowledge of nutrition, particularly as it relates to health and disease. Finally, other health professionals are finding themselves in positions that require them to provide direct nutritional counseling to patients and recognize a void in their training in this area. This book is an attempt to deal with the major issues in nutrition as they relate to human health and disease. It is designed as a textbook for undergraduate medical students and for students of other health professions and as a practical guide for house staff and practitioners as they deal with patients.

The book is organized in the same way as the nutrition course required of all first year medical and dental students at Columbia University College of Physicians and Surgeons. It is divided into four major parts: nutrition during various phases of the life cycle, such as pregnancy, infancy and childhood, adolescence, and old age; nutritional deficiencies, including calories, protein, fat, vitamins, and minerals; nutritional excess of the most important nutrients, covering in this context such diseases as obesity and atherosclerosis as well as the use and misuse of megadoses of vitamins and minerals; and diets both for the general public and for patients with specific diseases.

Although by no means all inclusive, the book covers what I believe are the major issues facing the public in general and health professionals in particular in the area of nutrition as it relates to human health and disease. It deals with the everyday questions people ask their health advisers as well as the role of nutrition in the management of such complicated disorders as diabetes, hypertension, atherosclerotic heart disease, renal disease, gastrointestinal disease, and cancer. It discusses not only the most commonly used diets but the indications for both enteral and parenteral nutrition and the practical approaches to implementing such therapy.

No single book can cover all of the topics discussed here in the kind of depth required for a complete mastery of each of the subjects. Hence, two types of judgment had to be made—which subjects to include and which to omit, and the relative importance of each particular subject. These judgments were made by me in consultation with others. It is for this reason and not because I consider myself an expert in all of these areas that the book was singly authored. However, single authorship of necessity introduces a certain amount of bias. In areas that are controversial I have tried to present both sides of the controversy but I have also tried to state clearly my own opinion, based sometimes on direct involvement in the field but more often on my own critical evaluation of the literature.

It is my sincere hope that this book will accelerate the trend toward including at least one course in nutrition in the training of every health professional.

I wish to express my appreciation to Professor John Dickerson of the University of Surrey for his critical review of the manuscript and his many thoughtful suggestions. In addition, I would like to thank Professor John Waterlow for providing access to the library of the London School of Hygiene and Tropical Medicine. My appreciation also goes to my wife Elaine for editing the manuscript.

MYRON WINICK

New York, New York
March 1980

CONTENTS

NUTRITION IN
HEALTH AND DISEASE

PART I
NUTRITION DURING THE LIFE CYCLE

1

NUTRITION DURING PREGNANCY

MATERNAL ADAPTATION

During pregnancy the mother's body undergoes a series of adaptations that create an environment optimal for fetal growth and that prepare her for the period of lactation to follow. The adaptations include a certain amount of weight gain independent of that due to the weight of the developing fetus. For example, early in pregnancy, while the placenta and fetus are still quite small, the size of the uterus begins to increase, breast tissue begins to develop, the volume of circulating blood expands, and "storage" fat is deposited deep within the mother's body. The uterus expands to accommodate the anticipated products of conception. The increased blood volume facilitates the flow of oxygen and nutrients across the placenta into the fetus as well as the removal of carbon dioxide and waste products. Breast enlargement and fat deposition prepare the mother for lactation, a period that will immediately follow delivery. Before the introduction of infant formulas, this particular adaptation of pregnancy was crucial to the survival of the infant.

If the maternal diet is inadequate either because insufficient food is available or because dietary restrictions have been imposed by well-meaning friends and relatives and sometimes even by well-meaning physicians, midwives, and nurses, fetal growth is impaired and the birth weight of the infant is reduced. The fetus is unable to extract the necessary nutrients to maintain optimal growth. This result might seem unlikely in view of the relatively large size of the mother when compared to that of the fetus. One might expect the mother to tap her own stores to supply the fetus. But

3

in fact this does not happen, and until recently there was no explanation for the mother's inability to mobilize her own reserves and transfer them to the fetus. In the last few years, we have begun to understand this apparent paradox.

Recent evidence both in animals and in humans suggests that inadequate nutrition, especially consumption of insufficient calories, will result in incomplete maternal adaptation to pregnancy. The expected increase in maternal blood volume will not take place in undernourished animals or humans. This, in turn, leads to a reduction in uterine and placental blood flow. As a result, the placenta itself will not grow properly and will not transfer nutrients adequately. Thus the process by which nutrients are actually passed to the fetus is imparied and hence even though these nutrients are available from maternal reserves they cannot reach the fetus in normal quantities. It is interesting to speculate about why such a state of affairs should exist. Why would fetal growth be sacrificed and maternal reserves be protected? The present view is that these reserves are essential for use during lactation. It is only when we view pregnancy and lactation as a continuum that we can see the "logic" in protecting the mother at the expense of fetal growth. Thus for optimal fetal growth and development, proper nutrition *during* pregnancy is extremely important.

WEIGHT GAIN

Until only a few years ago, rigid weight control during pregnancy was established medical practice. Recently, the Committee on Maternal Nutrition of the Food and Nutrition Board, National Research Council, as well as the Committee on Nutrition of the American College of Obstetrics and Gynecology, have recommended a weight gain of about 25 lb during the course of a normal pregnancy. Why have these recommendations for greater weight gain been made and what do they mean to the practicing physician?

Statistically, infant mortality and morbidity are much greater in low birth weight infants. Seventeen countries have lower infant mortality rates than the United States, and the major factor involved in this high mortality is our relatively high incidence of low birth weight infants.

The most powerful determinant of fetal birth weight is maternal weight gain during pregnancy. Statistically, the greater the maternal weight gain the bigger the infant at birth. This correlation holds for both affluent and impoverished populations. Maternal weight gain, in turn, is directly dependent on maternal diet during pregnancy.

The changes within the mother and the additional weight of the products of conception can account for the 25 lb that should be gained. During the first trimester these changes are accompanied by a minimal weight gain (1 to 2 kg). Thereafter, weight gain is linear, averaging 350 to 400 g/week. Such a course will result in a gain of about 10 to 12 kg by term. Figure 1 demonstrates the components of this weight gain.

During the second trimester it is the maternal compartment that adds weight (blood volume increase, uterine and breast growth, and fat storage). During the third trimester weight is rapidly added to the components of the fetal compartment (fetus, placenta, and amniotic fluid). Based on these considerations we can see that the correlation between maternal nutrition and birth weight is strongest during late pregnancy.

Adequate nutrition is important not only during pregnancy, since chronic undernutrition prior to pregnancy also will reduce birth weight. Thus prepregnant weight and weight gain during pregnancy exert independent and additive influences on birth weight. Together they account for almost all the variations at any given gestational age. Although most of the studies of outcome in human pregnancies have focused on birth weight, under-nutrition also reduces length, head circumference, and placental weight. Table 1 presents practical guidelines for assessing prepregnancy weight and weight gain during pregnancy.

The principal hazard facing the underweight patient is a low birth weight infant. For her, adequate weight gain during pregnancy is particu-larly important. What might appear unusual, however, is that the over-

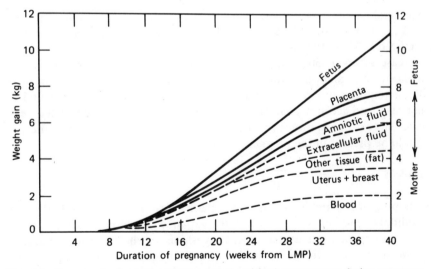

Figure 1. Components of weight gain in maternal and fetal compartment during pregnancy. (From R. M. Pitkin, in Schneider, 1977.)

Table 1.   Classification of weight and weight gain during pregnancy

Underweight	Prepregnant weight 10% or more below standard weight for height and age
Overweight	Prepregnant weight 20% or more above standard weight for height and age
Inadequate gain	Gain of 1 kg or less per month during second to third trimester
Excessive gain	Gain of 3 kg or more per month

weight obstetrical patient must also gain adequate weight during pregnancy to ensure a normal size infant. Admittedly the obese patient has a greater risk of developing chronic hypertensive vascular disease and diabetes mellitus, but restriction of weight gain during pregnancy to the extent of reaching parturition with a net loss does not reduce the incidence of these complications and will result in a lowering of birth weight.

NUTRIENT REQUIREMENTS DURING PREGNANCY

Calories

The total energy cost of pregnancy, calculated from the amounts of protein and fat accumulated by mother and fetus and the additional metabolism incurred by these tissues, amounts to approximately 75,000 kcal, or a daily increase of about 300 kcal. This represents about 15% above the recommended daily allowance for the nonpregnant mature "reference" woman. These requirements relate only to the increased needs of pregnancy and do not take into account such variables as physical activity, ambient temperature, or growth requirements of the mother unrelated to the pregnancy, as would be present in the pregnant adolescent.

Protein

The protein requirements during pregnancy have not been clearly defined. Additional protein is required for the expanded maternal plasma, uterus, and breasts, as well as for protein synthesis in the fetus and placenta. If we simply add up the amount of protein stored in these compartments we can calculate that 10 g/day of extra protein would be necessary in the diet. However, when nitrogen balance studies have been done, the actual protein requirement has always been shown to be two to three times that figure. This suggests that protein is stored in other depots such as skeletal muscle. As a result of these studies the present recommendations accept the higher figure. The recommended dietary allowance for protein for the pregnant woman has therefore been set as follows:

Mature woman	1.3 g/kg/day
Adolescent (age 15–18)	1.5 g/kg/day
Girl (under 15)	1.7 g/kg/day

Iron and Folate

Plasma volume increases progressively during early and middle pregnancy and levels off in the last few weeks before term. By this time the volume is 50% above the nonpregnant volume. By contrast, erythrocyte volume increases only 20% if no iron supplementation is given. Hence hemoglobin concentration will fall during pregnancy and anemia is very common. If iron is given, red cell volume will increase by 30%, suggesting that the limiting factor in erythropoiesis is availability of iron. The amount of elemental iron utilized by the increased maternal erythropoiesis is 500 mg. If we then add the 250 to 300 mg of iron needed for the fetus and placenta, the "iron requirement" of pregnancy is about 750 mg.

This requirement theoretically can be met by increasing dietary iron, utilizing maternal iron stores, or actually supplementing with iron. In most American women storage and diet combined will usually not be able to supply adequate amounts of iron. Therefore, routine iron supplementation during pregnancy is recommended. If 30 to 60 mg/day are given, iron deficiency anemia can be virtually eliminated as a complication of pregnancy.

Megaloblastic anemia due to folate deficiency was first recognized in a pregnant woman. The majority of cases in the United States are associated with pregnancy. Folate requirements increase during pregnancy not only because of the augmented maternal erythropoiesis that is occurring but also because of the requirements for adequate growth of the placenta and fetus. The recommended daily allowance for folate is 800 μg/day during pregnancy (twice the nonpregnant allowance).

Routine folate supplementation is controversial because the significance of low folate levels in the absence of anemia is not known. Some authorities use supplementation only when the dietary history suggests a low intake or when certain clinical conditions (e.g., chronic hemolytic anemia, multiple pregnancy, anticonvulsant drug therapy) cause an increased requirement. Others prefer routine folate supplementation. If vitamin supplementation is to be given, there is probably more reason to give folate than any other vitamin. This is especially true because recent survey data suggest that the amount of folate in most American diets may be marginal. Four hundred to eight hundred μg daily would be an appropriate supplementary amount.

Calcium and Vitamin D

The calcium content of the fetal skeleton averages 30 g, with most of the accumulation occurring during the last trimester. In addition, some evidence suggests that calcium is stored in the maternal skeleton during pregnancy, perhaps in anticipation of lactation needs. The recommended dietary allowance for calcium in pregnancy is 1200 mg, an increase of 400 mg over the allowance for the nonpregnant woman. This intake should provide adequate amounts, particularly in view of the adaptive ability to increase absorption and decrease excretion at times of increased need.

Deficient calcium intake during pregnancy can apparently result in osteomalacia in the mother, and there is radiographic evidence of decreased bone density in the infant. Vitamin D requirements do not appear to be increased markedly in pregnancy and the recommended dietary allowance is 400 IU/day for both pregnant and nonpregnant adults. Recent evidence suggests that in addition to its role in promoting a positive calcium balance during gestation, the vitamin may play a role in neonatal calcium homeostasis. Vitamin D and its metabolites cross the placenta freely and low plasma levels have been found in some instances of early neonatal hypocalcemia, suggesting that maternal vitamin D deficiency in late pregnancy may be responsible for this complication. At the opposite extreme, a possible association of maternal hypervitaminosis D and the severe form of infantile hypercalcemia is suggested by epidemiologic observations and animal studies.

Other Vitamins and Minerals

Virtually all other vitamins and minerals are needed in modestly increased amounts during pregnancy. Usually the levels required can be provided readily by diet. However, the practice of supplying routine supplementation is not dangerous as long as toxic overdoses are avoided, and supplementation should therefore be viewed as an option.

Summary

It should be clear that at present proper nutrition during pregnancy is extremely important to both the mother and the fetus. Therefore ensuring proper nutrition becomes a prime responsibility of the physician. Detailed dietary information should be obtained as part of the history. A complete physical examination requires a clinical assessment of nutritional status, and a height:weight ratio should be obtained for each patient. In addition, skinfold measurements to assess both muscle mass and adipose tissue mass should become a routine part of the physical examination. Careful observation for signs of any nutrient deficiency should be made. Finally, laboratory tests for anemia and urine analysis should be performed. During pregnancy, weight gain should, of course, be carefully monitored and if it is inadequate, dietary advice should be given. Iron should be routinely supplemented and folate supplementation at present should be optional but is recommended when intake data suggest a deficiency. Careful attention to meeting the daily nutrient requirements (Table 2) not only should ease the course of pregnancy but also will provide the best nutritional environment for the developing fetus.

Table 2. Recommended nutrient intake per day during pregnancy (mature woman)

Calories	2300
Protein	1.3 g/kg
Iron	30–60 mg
Folate	800 μg
Calcium	1200 mg
Vitamin D	400 IU

RECOMMENDED READING

Schneider, H. A., C. Anderson, and D. Coursin, Eds., *Nutritional Support of Medical Practice,* Harper and Row, New York, 1977, pp. 407–421.

Stein, Z. A., M. W. Susser, G. Saenger, and F. Marolla, *Famine and Human Development: The Dutch Hunger Winter of 1944/1945,* Oxford University Press, New York, 1975.

Winick, M., Ed., *Nutrition and Fetal Development,* Wiley, New York, 1974.

Winick, M., *Malnutrition and Brain Development,* Oxford University Press, New York, 1976.

2

INFANT FEEDING

An important new principle that is applicable to all aspects of child rearing, but is particularly important in the area of early nutrition, is the concept of imprinting. We now know that the early environment, including early nutritional practices, can cause changes in normal growth and development whose marks, or imprints, persist throughout life. For example, the caloric intake during the early growing period, while cells in various organs are still dividing, can alter the rate of cell division and result in an organ with fewer or greater than the expected number of cells. Thus severe under-nutrition may result in retarded cell division in the brain, and subsequently in a brain with a reduced number of cells. Conversely, overnutrition, especially excess caloric intake, may result in accelerated cell division in adipose tissue and in a permanently hypercellular adipose depot. This is associated in adult life with an extremely refractory kind of obesity. Less well studied, but perhaps of even greater health significance, is the relation between later atherosclerosis and early ingestion of cholesterol and saturated fat. What we know so far is that even in young adults found to have died of other causes, moderate fatty streaking and plaque formation can be found in arterial walls. Since high amounts of cholesterol and saturated fat in the diet constitute one major risk factor in atherosclerotic heart disease (see Chapter 13), concern has been mounting that the amount of these substances in the infant diet might in some way influence the later develop-ment of coronary heart disease.

Hence the well-trained physician must be concerned not only with the quantity but also with the quality of the infant diet. He must recommend a feeding pattern that takes into account the latest thinking in the areas of caloric requirement, percent of macronutrients, and amounts of micronutrients. Since requirements will vary at different ages, he must be aware of the dynamics of change as the infant grows.

NUTRIENT REQUIREMENTS

Table 1 sets forth the recommended daily allowance (RDA) for infants and young children. The requirements for protein and energy are listed but how that energy should be derived (the percent fat versus the percent carbohydrate) is left open. This is an expression more of our lack of knowledge than of our conviction that the source of energy is unimportant.

Table 1. Recommended daily dietary allowances (RDA)[a]

Nutrient	Age (years)		
	0–0.5	0.5–1.0	1–3
Energy (kcal)	117/kg	108/kg	1300
Protein (g)	2.2/kg	2.0/kg	23
Vitamin A (IU)	1400	2000	2000
Vitamin D (IU)	400	400	400
Vitamin E (IU)	4	5	7
Ascorbic acid (mg)	35	35	45
Folacin (μg)	30	45	100
Niacin (mg)	6	8	9
Riboflavin (mg)	0.4	0.6	0.8
Thiamin (mg)	0.3	0.5	0.7
Vitamin B_6 (mg)	0.3	0.6	0.9
Vitamin B_{12} (μg)	0.5	1.5	2.0
Calcium (mg)	360	540	800
Phosphorus (mg)	240	360	800
Iodine (μg)	40	50	70
Iron (mg)	10	15	15
Magnesium (mg)	50	70	150
Zinc (mg)	3	5	10

[a]The recommended dietary allowances are the amounts of essential nutrients considered by the Food and Nutrition Board to be adequate to meet the known nutritional needs of practically all healthy persons. Food and Nutrition Board, NAS-NRC, revised 1980.

The requirements for protein assume high quality protein, such as the casein or whey proteins usually found in breast milk. Again, nothing more specific is recommended since it is assumed that as long as all the essential amino acids are supplied (nine in the case of a young infant) the source is not important. This may not be entirely true, for we are beginning to learn that the types of protein may indeed be important and that protein mixtures resembling breast milk may be more efficiently utilized than other protein mixtures.

The requirements for vitamins and minerals have been calculated from the amounts necessary to prevent deficiency symptoms plus a "margin of safety" to cover those infants whose requirements may be higher. The method of setting these RDAs is necessarily imprecise, and although it is perhaps the best educated guess at the time the standards are being set, these allowances are constantly being revised as new information becomes available.

This method of arriving at recommended daily allowances has been criticized by certain groups, particularly a segment of the population that believes in higher requirements for vitamins and minerals. These groups assume that the requirements for optimal health may be different from those necessary to prevent deficiency symptoms and that the "margin of safety" is not nearly enough. There may well be a certain amount of truth in these criticisms but the problem is that we do not know how to define optimal health and we do know that excess amounts of certain vitamins and minerals can be extremely toxic. This is particularly true of vitamins A and D, and of calcium, phosphorus, and iodine. Until a more precise method of determining the optimal amount of each nutrient is found, the present system, though imperfect, seems to be the best available. However the physician should be aware of its shortcomings and should utilize new information as it appears.

Certain information that will necessitate changes and additions to the RDAs is already available. For example, essential fatty acid deficiency in infancy is now well recognized, and hence requirements for essential fatty acids will have to be set. From a practical standpoint this means that a certain amount of fat of mixed composition is necessary for optimal growth and development. Totally skimmed milk for an infant not receiving fat from other sources is, therefore, not recommended.

ASSESSMENT OF NUTRITIONAL STATUS

The most accurate index of adequate nutrition during the first year of life is "normal growth." The rate of growth is more sensitive than any other measurement to the total caloric and amino acid requirements of an infant.

In fact the studies in infants that originally defined those amino acids which were essential used the ability to support normal growth as their primary criterion. The most up to date height and weight curves are those derived from the recent HANES study and published by the Department of Health, Education, and Welfare.

Although most physicians are used to plotting height and weight versus age on growth charts, little attention has been paid to the actual composition of the weight being deposited. Recently we have become more and more aware of the importance of body composition in assessing whether an infant is growing properly and hence whether his nutrition is adequate. Standards of weight for height can be calculated from the weight and height curves. These should be used much more than they are. Such ratios are extremely important in suggesting whether the infant is depositing too much or too little fat tissue. Fat deposition can actually be measured more directly by using calipers and measuring triceps or subscapular skinfold thickness. Figures 1 and 2 show curves derived from such measurements for boys and girls during the first 18 months of life.

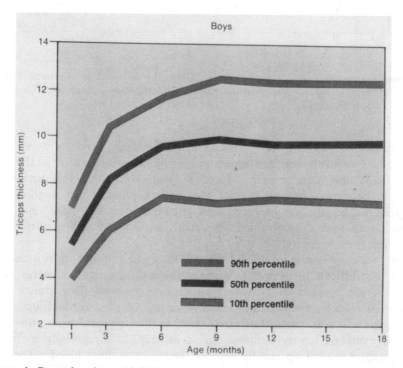

Figure 1. Range for triceps skinfold thickness in normal boys from 1 to 18 months. Taken from M. Winick, in *Year One: Nutrition, Growth, Health,* Ross Laboratories, Columbus, Ohio, 1975, p. 11.

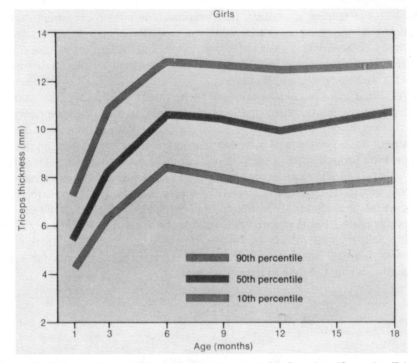

Figure 2. Range for triceps skinfold thickness in normal girls from 1 to 18 months. Taken from M. Winick, in *Year One: Nutrition, Growth, Health,* Ross Laboratories, Columbus, Ohio, 1975, p. 11.

Studies have shown that skinfold determinations, carefully done, are extremely accurate and can give a more precise estimation of total body fat than more cumbersome "research" methods. These measurements should become a routine part of the infant's physical examination, as routine as length, weight, and head circumference. They are relatively easy to do and a well-trained physician's assistant or office nurse can perform them accurately.

With a combination of careful dietary history and growth measurements it is not difficult to determine whether the requirements for energy and protein are being met. However, measurements other than growth are required to determine whether levels of certain of the micronutrients are adequate. Iron is particularly important in this respect, since iron deficiency anemia is very common during infancy. It is especially common if the child is growing rapidly because during such times blood volume is expanding at its greatest rate and hence new hemoglobin is being synthesized, requiring increased availability of iron. Breast milk, while low in total iron, has iron available in a more absorbable form than cow's milk or unfortified formula. Hence the breast fed infant rarely becomes iron deficient. In all infants, however, determination of iron status is an important part of the physician's responsibility. Iron status is determined most simply by measuring hemoglobin or hematocrit concentrations several times during the first two years of life. Although the experts do not agree completely on precise normal values, certainly a hemoglobin below 11 g after the first few weeks of life is unacceptable. Other tests, such as the serum ferritin test, have recently become available for more precise determination of iron status. At present, however, they are not available for routine clinical use. Any child who has had hemolytic disease during the neonatal period or who was premature at birth is particularly sensitive to developing subsequent iron deficiency anemia. Such children should be monitored extremely carefully and, as we shall see, their diets should be routinely supplemented with iron.

During the past few years, a number of pediatricians have begun to monitor the level of cholesterol in all of their patients. This procedure will identify those infants with a tendency to high values either for genetic reasons or because of a hyperresponse to exogenous cholesterol. Such infants can be placed on diets with lowered amounts of cholesterol and usually serum values will fall. The assessment of nutritional status is not difficult and should become a routine part of infant care. Table 2 outlines the ways in which a physician can efficiently determine the nutritional status of a young infant.

How should infants be fed in order to ensure adequate overall nutrition and optimal growth and development? The mother of a new infant and the physician caring for that infant have two major considerations to decide upon in relation to how to feed the child during the earliest stages of life: (1) whether to breast feed or bottle feed; (2) when and how to introduce solid foods. The first decision should be made before the infant is born so that the mother can be prepared for the initial feedings.

Table 2. Procedure for determining nutritional status

History	Type of formula; amount consumed or time spent on nursing; other foods consumed, especially those high in saturated fat or low in iron
Anthropomorphic measurements	All visits; height, weight, head circumference, subscapular or triceps fatfold thickness
Laboratory	Hemoglobin, hematocrit, and serum cholesterol at 3 months and 1 year

BREAST VERSUS BOTTLE FEEDING

Breast milk has been the natural method of infant feeding throughout the ages. All mammals breast feed and the composition of their breast milk has evolved in a highly individualized manner to meet the needs of both the infant and the mother of a particular species. The process of lactation is one during which a number of changes occur, beginning in late pregnancy and culminating in the synthesis and secretion of milk. We do not know the long-term consequences to the mother of artificially shutting off these mechanisms after the infant is born. For example, the metabolic demands of lactation and hence the nutritional requirements during this period are much greater than during pregnancy. To prepare for this all mammals, including the human, deposit fat tissue around deep organs during pregnancy, to be utilized during lactation. The average mother will deposit 2 to 4 kg (5 to 10 lb) of fat in this manner. Thus from a practical standpoint, weight loss after pregnancy to reach prepregnancy weight is much more difficult if a mother is not breast feeding. The breast feeding mother will gradually consume the excess fat during the metabolic processes involved in milk synthesis. During lactation, then, the mother should consume a higher caloric diet than during pregnancy. At present the recommended dietary allowance for calories is 2600 kcal/day during lactation. This is best achieved by increasing the quantity of all three major nutrients: protein, carbohydrate, and fat.

Human breast milk is highly adapted for the human infant and is an almost complete source of all required nutrients. If the mother is well nourished, the infant will grow adequately on breast milk alone for the first 6 months of life. Human milk is a relatively low protein milk, containing approximately one-fourth the concentration of protein in cow's milk and one-tenth to one-fifteenth the protein content of milk of certain carnivores such as the fox and the dog. This is due to the relatively slow rate of growth of the human infant during the nursing period when compared to these other species. By contrast, human milk contains approximately the same fat content as cow's milk and somewhat more carbohydrate in the form of lactose than cow's milk. In addition, human milk protein differs qualitatively from cow's milk protein. The latter is almost entirely casein whereas the former is made up of equal amounts of casein and whey protein (mainly lactalbumin). This composition is in part related to the ability of the gastrointestinal tract of the human infant and the young calf to handle these particular proteins. In addition, lactalbumin contains greater amounts of the sulfur-containing amino acids, which may be essential during infancy. Although infant formulas that will simulate human milk can be constructed, they do not duplicate the actual composition of the protein or the fat present in human milk.

Human milk is rich in certain other nutrients required by the growing infant. For example, the average liter of human milk contains 43 mg of vitamin C in comparison to about 20 mg in a liter of cow's milk. With the exception perhaps of vitamin D, the young infant's dietary requirements are met by breast milk in a form that is most efficient for its body to absorb and utilize. Recent evidence suggests that the vitamin D content in human milk may be much greater than previously thought. The vitamin D is in a water soluble form and has hence been overlooked when the fat fraction was examined. This water soluble vitamin D fraction, when fed to young rats, has shown antirachitic activity. Whether this is true in the human infant is not yet known.

Breast milk offers advantages other than those based on nutrient content. The placentas of certain mammals will allow passage of the immunoglobin IgG during late gestation. In those mammals, including the human, the milk contains very little IgG and IgA is the predominant form of antibody found in both colostrum and milk. By contrast, in those mammals such as the cow, who do not transmit IgG, the predominant antibody type in the milk is IgG. Again, we can see pregnancy and lactation acting as a continuum in preparing the infant for external survival. The IgA in human milk probably offers protection from bacterial invasion at the surface of the gastrointestinal tract. In addition to antibodies, human milk transmits maternal macrophages capable of producing antibody and programmed into the maternal immune system, offering the infant protection from a variety of infections. Still another property of breast feeding that may be advantageous to the newborn is a factor in colostrum which has recently been described to stimulate the growth of the gastrointestinal tract. Although these experiments have been done only in animals, if confirmed in humans they could have important implications.

A final advantage of breast feeding is that the quantity taken in is controlled by the infant's satiety mechanisms rather than being determined by a preexisting figure in the mother's mind. It has been demonstrated recently that bottle fed babies consuming a formula of identical caloric content to human milk gain more weight during the first year of life than breast fed infants. This is no doubt due to the mother's desire to drain the bottle dry. In view of our concern about the early genesis of obesity, this increased weight gain may not be desirable. Table 3 summarizes the advantages of breast feeding.

The major advantage of bottle feeding is said to be convenience. I am not sure why it is more convenient to mix carefully a number of constituents

Table 3.   Advantages of breast feeding

Nutrition	Higher percentage of lactalbumin
	Richer in sulfur-containing amino acids
	More easily digestible
	Qualitatively different fat content (may or may not be important)
	Higher levels of certain vitamins (vitamin C and possibly D)
	Iron in an easily available form
Immunological	Colostrum richer in certain antibodies (IgA content higher)
	Contains maternal macrophages
Other	Infant controls own intake (reduces possibility of overfeeding)
	Colostrum may contain gut growth factor (animal data only)

and prepare a series of sterile formulas than to put a child to the breast. I am not even sure why the "modern" infant formula preparations are more "convenient" than breast feeding. How this notion took hold is difficult to understand, but it is extremely prevalent in our population. This can be appreciated simply by noting that 60% of our population never breast feed and 80% do not breast feed beyond 3 months of age. Thus formula feeding has become the rule rather than the exception and the physician, while attempting to change this trend, must be able to counsel the mother for efficient formula feeding. If evaporated milk is used, it must be suitably diluted to reduce the content of total solids and the caloric density as well as the protein content. In order to bring the protein concentration into the range of breast milk, caloric density will be lowered too much. Hence carbohydrate, usually in the form of dextromaltose, is added to reach the desired calorie concentration of 20 cal/oz. Commercially prepared formulas have already done all of this and one simply adds water or gives the formula which comes "ready to feed." In most prepared formulas the source of carbohydrate is lactose, the same as in breast milk. The source of protein is casein, prepared from cow's milk, and the fat content is more unsaturated and lower in cholesterol than the fat in human milk. Most prepared formulas are fortified with the recommended dietary allowances for most nutrients, and many even contain added iron. Thus, although they do not reproduce human milk in all particulars (primarily in the type of protein and fat), prepared formulas have been shown to supply an adequate total source of nutrition during early life. The major problem that must be impressed on the mother is that the feeding of any formula from a bottle will provide the temptation to overfeed. This should be discouraged. Another practice to discourage is propping the bottle into the infant's mouth and allowing him to suck himself to sleep. This exposes the erupting teeth to relatively high carbohydrate concentrations and may provide the conditions for the development of dental caries.

INTRODUCTION OF SOLID FOODS

The introduction of solid foods should be the beginning of a prolonged process by which the infant goes through a smooth transition from breast feeding to the family's regular diet. Weaning is usually begun gradually in the second 6 months of life. The trend toward artificial feeding of infants has brought with it a trend for earlier and earlier introduction of solid foods. One study found that by 1 month of age 67% of infants were taking solid foods and by 2 months 96% were already on solid foods. In general, the feeding of solid foods has not been as a replacement for formula but has been *in addition* to formula, resulting in an increase in calories consumed. Another study found that mean energy intake at 6 weeks of age was 135 kcal/kg and that weight gain was excessive. Still other studies reveal that by 3 months of age most infants in the United States are consuming an excess of almost all nutrients.

Given the tendency to consume excess calories and other nutrients, early introduction of solid foods, especially those of high caloric density, should be discouraged. The primary reason for this is a fear of inducing early obesity (see Chapter 12). I see no real need for solid foods before 4 months of age and I find no data to convince me that introducing solid foods will placate a "fussy" infant. At 4 months solid foods can be introduced slowly as a *replacement* for breast milk or formula. The caloric density and nutrient content of the particular foods should be known so that their contribution to the total dietary intake can be calculated. At this age it makes no difference whether commercially prepared or home prepared weaning foods are used. Since iron is often in low supply if the infant's diet is not being supplemented, fortified cereals might be the first solid foods introduced. (A complete discussion of iron requirements and deficiency is given in Chapter 10). If serum cholesterol levels are high, foods rich in cholesterol, primarily eggs, may be deferred until later.

Vitamin D supplementation is desirable if the infant is being maintained entirely on breast milk. Most infant formulas contain vitamin D in adequate amounts. After the infant is on a varied diet of solid foods (9 to 12 months of age) these supplements can be discontinued.

In summary, two major decisions must be made when determining how best to feed an infant during the first year of life: whether to breast or bottle feed, and when to introduce solid foods. Breast feeding has nutritional advantages, immunological advantages, and other advantages, as shown in Table 3, and should be encouraged. If bottle feeding is used, the tendency to overfeed should be resisted and the "propping" of bottles discouraged. Finally, the introduction of solid foods should be delayed until at least 4 months of age and then introduced slowly.

RECOMMENDED READING

Brown, R. E., Breast Feeding in Modern Times, *Am. J. Clin. Nutr.*, **26**, 556 (1973).

Committee on Nutrition, American Academy of Pediatrics, Statement on Iron Supplementation for Infants, in Committee on Nutrition, *Collected Reprints 1967-1977*, American Academy of Pediatrics, Evanston, Ill., p. 163.

Drizizen, S., The Importance of Nutrition in Tooth Development, *J. Sch. Health*, **43**, 114 (1973).

Fomon, S. J., *Protein in Infant Nutrition*, 2nd ed., Saunders, Philadelphia, 1974.

Jelliffe, D. B., and E. F. Patrice, Lactation, Conception, and the Nutrition of the Nursing Mother and Child, *J. Pediat.*, **81**, 829 (1972).

Kennel, W. R., and T. R. Dawber, Atherosclerosis as a Pediatric Problem, *J. Pediat.*, **80**, 544 (1972).

McClaren, D. S., and D. Burman, *Textbook of Pediatric Nutrition*, Churchill Livingston, Edinburgh, 1976.

Nutrition Committee of the Canadian Pediatric Society and the Committee on Nutrition, American Academy of Pediatrics, Statement on Breast Feeding, *Pediatrics*, **62**, 591 (1978).

Theuer, R. C., Iron Undernutrition in Infancy, *Clin. Pediat.*, **13**, 522 (1974).

3

NUTRITION DURING ADOLESCENCE

The period of adolescence, accompanied by its profound changes in growth rates, body composition, and marked physiologic and endocrine changes, is a time of life when the individual is at particular nutritional risk. And yet we really know very little about the actual nutritional requirements during adolescence and our recommendations at present are based on only fragmentary evidence. In addition, the changes that occur during adolescence are markedly different in the two sexes, suggesting that requirements may also differ. The few guidelines we have, however, often do not differentiate between the sexes for certain nutrient requirements.

During the middle school years boys and girls grow in a comparable manner, gaining 2 to 3 kg/year in weight and approximately 1 cm/year in height. The adolescent growth spurt begins earlier in girls than in boys, and at about 10 years of age girls begin to grow more rapidly. The peak growth velocity for females precedes the actual entry into puberty and occurs between 10 and 12.5 years. During this period the average girl will gain 8.3 kg/year and grow 8.3 cm/year. In boys, the growth spurt begins later, beginning at 12 years and continues until 14 years of age. During this period he will gain approximately 9 kg/year and grow 9.5 cm/year. Hence men are taller than women because they enter adolescence later (gaining 5 to 6 cm in the preceding 2 years) and because they grow more than girls during the adolescent spurt. In general, children entering adolescence early tend to be shorter adults whereas those entering late tend to be taller.

vision impairment halts with stop in height increase

21

Marked changes in body composition also occur during the adolescent period. Males deposit proportionally more lean body tissue and skeletal mass whereas females deposit proportionally more fat. Thus a boy reaching 180 cm in height will have about 9 kg of total body fat; a girl of the same height will have about 20 kg of adipose tissue. These differences are reflected in the triceps skinfold thickness. Whether plotted against stage of puberty or chronological age, the thickness increases during puberty in girls and actually decreases in boys. There are data which suggest that this deposition of fat during adolescence may be due to actual increases in the number of adipocytes within the various adipose depots.

Other changes that occur during adolescence would suggest an increased need for specific nutrients. For example, the rapid increase in body size will be accompanied by a rapid increase in blood volume, suggesting an increased need for iron. In addition, the onset of menstruation in the female will again increase the iron requirement as a result of blood loss.

What, then, are the nutritional requirements of the adolescent boy and girl and how can they best be met? Energy requirements increase to support growth and are maximal during the growth spurt. In boys 2800 to 3000 kcal/day are recommended between ages 11 and 18; in girls, 2400 kcal/day between ages 11 and 14 and 2100 kcal/day between 15 and 18. These figures are calculated based on theoretically estimated needs to achieve the desired growth rates and changes in body composition rather than by any direct measurements. The protein requirements obviously increase during this period of intense anabolism. Boys 11 to 14 require 45 g and boys 15 to

Table 1. Food and Nutrition Board, National Academy of Sciences—National

	Age (years)	Weight (kg)	Weight (lb)	Height (cm)	Height (in.)	Energy (kcal)	Protein (g)	Vitamin A Activity (RE)[a]	Vitamin A Activity (IU)	Vitamin D (IU)	Vitamin E Activity[b] (IU)
Males	11–14	45	99	157	62	2700	45	1000	5000	400	12
	15–18	66	145	176	69	2800	56	1000	5000	400	15
Females	11–14	46	101	157	62	2200	46	800	4000	400	12
	15–18	55	120	163	64	2100	46	800	4000	400	12
Pregnant						+300	+30	1000	5000	600	15
Lactating						+500	+20	1200	6000	600	15

[a] Retinol equivalents.
[b] Total vitamin E activity; estimated as 80% alpha tocopherol and 20% other tocopherols.
[c] The folacin allowances refer to dietary sources as determined by *Lactobacillus casei* assay. Pure forms of folacin may be effective in doses less than one-fourth of the recommended dietary allowance.

18 require 56 g. In girls the requirement is somewhat different—46 g and 46 g, respectively. This relatively high protein requirement can represent a problem in feeding the adolescent, who often has strange eating patterns which result in the ingestion of a high carbohydrate and relatively low protein diet.

As mentioned earlier, iron requirements increase during this period of life. The recent ten state nutrition survey in the United States showed a high prevalence of iron deficiency in this age group. An unexpected finding was that the prevalence was greater in boys than in girls. The RDA for iron is 18 mg/day in this age group, which is the highest for any period of life except pregnancy. This requirement is difficult to meet from diet alone without consumption of liberal amounts of red meats or fortified foods. Adolescents on vegetarian diets may be particularly susceptible to iron deficiency and probably should receive oral iron supplementation.

Table 1 indicates the recommended dietary allowances for most nutrients. It can be seen that requirements for literally all nutrients are very high during this period of life.

How can we achieve these requirements in the adolescent? Many adolescents, like our modern adult population, are very concerned with nutrition. This concern, coupled with the curiosity that is common at this time of life, may lead to the "trying out" of all sorts of diets. Thus many adolescents experiment with vegetarian diets, organic foods, macrobiotic diets, and so on. Although these diets are considered in Chapter 17, it should be pointed out here that discussing the diet with the adolescent patient, and carefully

Research Council recommended daily dietary allowance, revised 1980

	Water-Soluble Vitamins						Minerals					
Ascorbic Acid (mg)	Folacin[c] (μg)	Niacin[d] (mg)	Riboflavin (mg)	Thiamin (mg)	Vitamin B$_6$ (mg)	Vitamin B$_{12}$ (μg)	Calcium (mg)	Phosphorus (mg)	Iodine (μg)	Iron (mg)	Magnesium (mg)	Zinc (mg)
50	400	18	1.6	1.4	1.8	3.0	1200	1200	150	18	350	15
60	400	18	1.7	1.4	2.0	3.0	1200	1200	150	18	400	15
50	400	15	1.3	1.1	1.8	3.0	1200	1200	150	18	300	15
60	400	14	1.3	1.1	2.0	3.0	1200	1200	150	18	300	15
+20	800	+2	+0.3	+0.4	+0.6	4.0	1600	1600	+25	18+[e]	450	20
+40	500	+5	+0.5	+0.5	+0.5	4.0	1600	1600	+50	18	450	25

[d] Although allowances are expressed as niacin, on the average 1 mg of niacin is derived from each 60 mg of dietary tryptophan.

[e] This increased requirement cannot be met by ordinary diets; therefore the use of supplemental iron is recommended.

finding out what he or she is actually eating, will allow the physician to suggest minor modifications or certain types of supplementation that can materially improve the intake of important nutrients. For example, vegetarian diets may be quite different. The strict vegetarian who eats no meat or meat products will have a low protein intake unless he consumes certain types of legumes. Just adding soy beans and certain kinds of nuts to such a diet can increase the protein intake considerably. In addition, iron and vitamin B_{12} will be low, and suggesting supplementation or the use of fortified cereals may alleviate the problem. By contrast, the "vegetarian diet" which allows eggs, milk, and milk products does not need special advice in regard to protein and vitamin B_{12}. Iron, however, should still be supplemented. Natural or organic diets are usually nutritionally sound, although often expensive. What is important is not the name of the diet but what is actually consumed by the adolescent.

Most of the potential nutritional problems in this population can be avoided by proper advice without radically changing the diet and the eating patterns of the adolescent. This is very important, because a radical change in diet is unlikely to be accepted. It is important to discuss these dietary modifications with the adolescent rather than impose a set of rigid rules. Finally, this may be a good opportunity to discuss general nutritional principles with a receptive individual.

Some adolescents will have erratic and sometimes even bizarre eating patterns. Soft drinks, potato chips, and candy bars may constitute the mainstays of their food intake. Here, radical change is in order, but the importance of such a change must be explained. Several alternative approaches should be discussed. The decision as to how to change should be one between the physician and the adolescent. This type of therapy cannot simply be prescribed.

Recently we have been seeing a specific situation in adolescent girls which imposes a major additional nutritional stress. Pregnancy has been occurring more and more frequently in this age group and at younger and younger ages. The nutritional requirements are greater in this group of growing pregnant adolescents than in any other group of individuals. If they breast feed, these requirements become even greater. Table 1 shows the increased requirements for pregnancy and lactation, which must be added to the requirements for adolescence. This group by its very nature constitutes a high risk population during pregnancy and strict medical management including dietary management is mandatory (see Chapter 1). Breast feeding should be encouraged in adolescents as in other women and dietary intake should be increased accordingly. Iron and vitamins should be supplemented in the pregnant adolescent, since it is very difficult to meet the requirements by diet alone.

In summary, the period of adolescence is a time when major changes in body composition take place. These changes are accompanied by rapid growth and physiologic and behavioral alterations. Nutrient requirements change and dietary habits often change as well. Unfortunately the change in dietary habits is often dictated by factors other than the requirement for nutrients. Sometimes, in fact, these changes proceed in opposite directions. The physician should be aware of the special needs of the adolescent and must take into account the adolescent "life style" in order to achieve these needs. Nutritionally this can best be done by explaining the problem and offering the adolescent as many alternatives as possible.

RECOMMENDED READING

Brasel, J. A., in M. Winick, Ed., *Nutritional Disorders of American Women,* Wiley, New York, 1977, pp. 53-65.

Cheek, D., *Human Growth,* Lea and Febiger, Philadephia, 1968.

Heald, F. P., Ed., *Nutrition and Growth,* Appleton-Century-Crofts, New York, 1969.

Heyden, S., W. DeMaria, S. Barbee, and M. Morris, Weight Reduction in Adolescents, *Nutr. Metab.,* **15**, 45 (1973).

Huenemann, R. A., A Review of Teenage Nutrition, *U.S. Health Ser. Rep.,* **87**, 823 (1973).

King, J. C., S. H. Cohenour, D. H. Calloway, and H. N. Jacobson, Assessment of Nutritional Status of Teenage Pregnant Girls, *Am. J. Clin. Nutr.,* **25**, 916 (1972).

Webb, T. E., and F. A. Oski, Iron Deficiency Anemia and Scholastic Achievement in Young Adolescents, *J. Pediat.,* **82**, 827 (1973).

4

NUTRITION AND THE ELDERLY

More than 20 million Americans are 65 years old or older. We have in the United States 25,000 nursing homes containing a million and a half beds—more nursing home beds than hospital beds. The population of senior citizens is the fastest growing population in America. Thus the "problem" of aging, if we can call it that, is increasing in magnitude. This increase, of course, is partly due to improvements in health care, which are allowing people to live longer. If we succeed in many of our goals, such as reducing the incidence of heart disease and cancer, we will increase the number of our senior citizens even more. Thus, we have within our society, as well as in many other so-called advanced societies, what has become a contradiction that is often difficult to deal with; that is, more old people and, therefore, more problems of the elderly.

There are two ways in which one may deal with this problem: (1) by reducing the burdens that the elderly must bear and (2) by curtailing the process during the early and middle years that leads to the physiologic state that we define as "old age." In a sense, we must seek ways not of slowing but of actually changing the aging process, and methods of structuring the environment of those who reach old age to provide them with optimal health and well-being. Nutrition is an important component of both of these approaches.

From a nutritional standpoint the most important physiologic changes that occur during the aging process relate to the renal, gastrointestinal, and neuromuscular-skeletal systems. Renal function deteriorates with age. In humans, the renal flow and glomerular filtration rate decline with age as do the T_m for glucose and the T_m for PAH. In addition, the ability to form either a concentrated or a dilute urine is impaired. In rats, there is an actual decline in the number of nephrons.

Gastrointestinal function also deteriorates with age. The ability of parietal cells to secrete hydrochloric acid declines and in general, there is a reduction in the secretory ability of the digestive glands. Xylose absorption is normal until 80 years of age, whereas calcium absorption decreases beyond 65 years of age.

Thus certain digestive and absorptive functions are impaired with aging, whereas others are not.

Motor function also declines. Generalized weakness is probably due to both a decline in the number of functioning muscle fibers and a decrease in the actual strength of the contractile process itself.

Certain changes in body composition also occur during aging. Bone loss, beginning in the fifth decade, is almost universal. This process proceeds almost twice as fast in women as in men. Although it has been generally believed that there is a loss in lean body mass and an increase in the adipose tissue mass with age, the data have been gathered in cross-sectional studies. Recent data from longitudinal studies (i.e., collected on the same patient over a period of time) suggest that lean body mass does not decline with age but rather that individuals with a smaller lean body mass tend to live longer.

The changes outlined above suggest the need for careful evaluation of nutritional requirements for the elderly especially in relation to certain specific nutrients. For example, the decrease in muscle mass suggests that protein and amino acid requirements may change with age. The reduced calcium absorption coupled with bone resorption suggests that calcium and phosphorus requirements be reevaluated. The decreased secretion of hydrochloric acid coupled with general gastric atrophy suggests an increase in the iron and perhaps vitamin B_{12} requirements. Careful research aimed at determining requirements of most nutrients specifically for the elderly is just beginning. At present, neither current United States nor international dietary allowances have included separate recommendations for a single nutrient for the elderly.

The caloric requirements of the elderly are lower than those of the younger adult, partly because of the decreased activity of older people and probably also because of a decrease in basal requirements. The exact amount of this reduction has not been clearly determined, but the recommended daily allowances (eighth edition, 1974) proposes about a 10% reduction after the age of 50.

Nor have the protein requirements of the elderly been precisely worked out. In humans, the amount of total body protein synthesized daily declines with age. In addition, the relative amounts of protein synthesized by various

Table 1.   Recommended dietary allowances, revised 1980 Food and Nutrition Board,

Age and Sex Group	Weight		Height		Protein	Fat-soluble Vitamins		
						Vitamin A	Vitamin D	Vitamin E
	kg	lb	cm	in.	g	μg R.E. [b]	μg [c]	mg αT.E. [d]
Infants								
0.0–0.5 yr	6	13	60	24	kg. × 2.2	420	10	3
0.5–1.0 yr	9	20	71	28	kg. × 2.0	400	10	4
Children								
1–3 yr	13	29	90	35	23	400	10	5
4–6 yr	20	44	112	44	30	500	10	6
7–10 yr	28	62	132	52	34	700	10	7
Males								
11–14 yr	45	99	157	62	45	1000	10	8
15–18 yr	66	145	176	69	56	1000	10	10
19–22 yr	70	154	177	70	56	1000	7.5	10
23–50 yr	70	154	178	70	56	1000	5	10
51 + yr	70	154	178	70	56	1000	5	10
Females								
11–14 yr	46	101	157	62	46	800	10	8
15–18 yr	55	120	163	64	46	800	10	8
19–22 yr	55	120	163	64	44	800	7.5	8
23–50 yr	55	120	163	64	44	800	5	8
51 + yr	55	120	163	64	44	800	5	8
Pregnancy					+30	+200	+5	+2
Lactation					+20	+400	+5	+3

[a] The allowances are intended to provide for individual variations among most normal persons as they live in the United States under usual environmental stresses. Diets should be based on a variety of common foods in order to provide other nutrients for which human requirements have been less well defined.

[b] Retinol equivalents; 1 retinol equivalent = 1 μg retinol or 6 μg β-carotene.

[c] As cholecalciferol: 10 μg cholecalciferol = 400 IU vitamin D.

[d] α tocopherol equivalents: 1 mg d-α-tocopherol = 1 α T.E.

[e] 1 N.E. (niacin equivalent) = 1 mg niacin or 60 mg dietary tryptophan.

[f] The folacin allowances refer to dietary sources as determined by *Lactobacillus casei* assay after treatment with enzymes

organs is redistributed. Visceral tissue makes a greater over-all contribution to total body protein synthesis in the elderly than in the young adult. From these observations one is tempted to predict that the total protein requirement for the elderly should be less per unit of body weight. However, actual measurements of protein requirements, using a variety of techniques, suggest that the minimum protein needs of healthy adults do not change significantly with advancing age. On the basis of current knowledge, the recommended intake for healthy males is 56 g and for females it is 46 g. This amount appears to be adequate for most healthy elderly individuals.

Even less is known about amino acid requirements than about total protein requirements. Preliminary data suggest that the requirements of the elderly for the amino acids threonine and tryptophan are similar to those for young adults when expressed per unit of body weight. Nothing is known about the other amino acids.

National Academy of Sciences-National Research Council[a]

Water-soluble Vitamins							Minerals					
Vitamin C	Thiamin	Ribo-flavin	Niacin	Vitamin B6	Folacin[f]	Vitamin B12	Calcium	Phos-phorus	Mag-nesium	Iron	Zinc	Iodine
← mg →			mg N.E.[e]	mg	← μg →		← mg →					μg
35	0.3	0.4	6	0.3	30	0.5[g]	360	240	50	10	3	40
35	0.5	0.6	8	0.6	45	1.5	540	360	70	15	5	50
45	0.7	0.8	9	0.9	100	2.0	800	800	150	15	10	70
45	0.9	1.0	11	1.3	200	2.5	800	800	200	10	10	90
45	1.2	1.4	16	1.6	300	3.0	800	800	250	10	10	120
50	1.4	1.6	18	1.8	400	3.0	1200	1200	350	18	15	150
60	1.4	1.7	18	2.0	400	3.0	1200	1200	400	18	15	150
60	1.5	1.7	19	2.2	400	3.0	800	800	350	10	15	150
60	1.4	1.6	18	2.2	400	3.0	800	800	350	10	15	150
60	1.2	1.4	16	2.2	400	3.0	800	800	350	10	15	150
50	1.1	1.3	15	1.8	400	3.0	1200	1200	300	18	15	150
60	1.1	1.3	14	2.0	400	3.0	1200	1200	300	18	15	150
60	1.1	1.3	14	2.0	400	3.0	800	800	300	18	15	150
60	1.0	1.2	13	2.0	400	3.0	800	800	300	18	15	150
60	1.0	1.2	13	2.0	400	3.0	800	800	300	10	15	150
+20	+0.4	+0.3	+2	+0.6	+400	+1.0	+400	+400	+150	[h]	+5	+25
+40	+0.5	+0.5	+5	+0.5	+100	+1.0	+400	+400	+150	[h]	+10	+50

("conjugases") to make polyglutamyl forms of the vitamin available to the test organism.

[g] The RDA for vitamin B12 in infants is based on average concentration of the vitamin in human milk. The allowances after weaning are based on energy intake (as recommended by the American Academy of Pediatrics) and consideration of other factors, such as intestinal absorption.

[h] The increased requirement during pregnancy cannot be met by the iron content of habitual American diets or by the existing iron stores of many women; therefore, the use of 30 to 60 mg supplemental iron is recommended. Iron needs during lactation are not substantially different from those of nonpregnant women, but continued supplementation of the mother for 2 to 3 months after parturition is advisable in order to replenish stores depleted by pregnancy.

Despite the limited data available, decisions about protein and amino acid requirements for the elderly must be made. Tentatively, I would recommend that protein intake for the elderly consist of amounts adequate to meet the *minimum* daily requirement of the healthy young adult but not a great deal more than this. In addition, the protein should be supplied in a form that is rich in the essential amino acids and easily digestible. Thus, fish, soft cheese, lean meats, and fowl, as well as certain vegetable proteins, would be good choices. Since, as we have noted, hydrochloric acid in the stomach may not be secreted properly and the intrinsic factor may be low, the elderly may be more prone to anemia due to both poor iron absorption and poor absorption of vitamin B12. Therefore, foods rich in iron and vitamin B12 are indicated. These include red meat, liver, and fortified cereals. Requirements for other vitamins and minerals have not been established for the elderly; therefore, we can only provide what is

Table 2.   Estimated safe and adequate daily dietary intakes of additional selected

Age Group	Vitamins			Trace Elements[b]	
	Vitamin K	Biotin	Pantothenic Acid	Copper	Manganese
	← μg →		← mg →		
Infants					
0.0–0.5 yr	12	35	2	0.5–0.7	0.5–0.7
0.5–1.0 yr	10–20	50	3	0.7–1.0	0.7–1.0
Children and adolescents					
1–3 yr	15–30	65	3	1.0–1.5	1.0–1.5
4–6 yr	20–40	85	3–4	1.5–2.0	1.5–2.0
7–10 yr	30–60	120	4–5	2.0–2.5	2.0–3.0
11 + yr	50–100	100–200	4–7	2.0–3.0	2.5–5.0
Adults	70–140	100–200	4–7	2.0–3.0	2.5–5.0

[a]From Recommended Dietary Allowances, Revised 1980. Food and Nutrition Board, National Academy of Sciences—National Research Council. Because there is less information on which to base allowances, these figures are not given in the main table of the RDAs and are provided here in the form of ranges of recommended

adequate for the young adult. Older people, however, may be chronically deficient in calcium.

Two diseases that are quite common in the elderly, osteoporosis and periodontal disease, may be associated in part with chronic calcium deficiency. There are two schools of thought about the nature of these diseases.

One group of investigators believes that they are two different diseases, osteoporosis being a slowly progressing degenerative disease of bone, and periodontal disease being a chronic infection of the gums with erosion of the underlying bone, loosening, and finally loss of teeth. A second group of investigators feels that they are both the same disease arising from a chronic, long-term calcium deficiency, which slowly drains both the long bones and the jaw bones and results in a propensity toward long bone fractures and loss of teeth from their bony sockets.

Both groups agree that calcium treatment alone will do little for the patient with osteoporosis. However, those espousing the chronic calcium deficiency etiology believe that calcium supplementation before osteoporosis develops will prevent or at least delay the process. They feel that the recommended dietary allowance is much too low and that adults should take in a minimum of 1 g of calcium daily and preferably more than that.

vitamins and minerals [a]

Trace Elements [b]				Electrolytes		
Fluoride	Chromium	Selenium	Molyb-denum	Sodium	Potassium	Chloride
← mg →						
0.1–0.5	0.01–0.04	0.01–0.04	0.03–0.06	115– 350	350– 925	275– 700
0.2–1.0	0.02–0.06	0.02–0.06	0.04–0.08	250– 750	425–1275	400–1200
0.5–1.5	0.02–0.08	0.02–0.08	0.05–0.1	325– 975	550–1650	500–1500
1.0–2.5	0.03–0.12	0.03–0.12	0.06–0.15	450–1350	775–2325	700–2100
1.5–2.5	0.05–0.2	0.05–0.2	0.1 –0.3	600–1800	1000–3000	925–2775
1.5–2.5	0.05–0.2	0.05–0.2	0.15–0.5	900–2700	1525–4575	1400–4200
1.5–4.0	0.05–0.2	0.05–0.2	0.15–0.5	1100–3300	1875–5625	1700–5100

intakes.

[b] Since the toxic levels for many trace elements may be only several times usual intakes, the upper levels for the trace elements given in this table should not be habitually exceeded.

In addition, based on experiments with periodontal disease in horses and on limited trials in humans with periodontal disease, this group feels that calcium therapy in high doses will reverse the process in the jaw bones and lead to the healing of the periodontal tissues and strengthening of the teeth within their sockets.

My own feeling, based on my understanding of the data, is that osteoporosis may be due to in part to a chronic calcium deficiency because of the low intake of calcium by modern society. (See Chapter 10 for a detailed discussion of calcium metabolism.) I would therefore recommend that foods rich in calcium be eaten during adult life as well as during childhood and that patients who are middle-aged and who have symptoms or x-ray findings of osteoporosis be supplemented with 1 g/day of calcium in the form of gluconate. Although I am not convinced that this will prevent progression of the disease, I feel that the risk of this form of prophylaxis is minimal and the potential benefits are high enough to warrant this approach.

With periodontal disease, the data are difficult to interpret. Currently, I feel that this is a disease of multiple etiology and that some forms may respond to calcium treatment. Since this treatment has been reported in some cases to be of considerable benefit, with objective changes in the x-ray

Table 3. Mean heights and weights and recommended energy intake [a]

Age and Sex Group	Weight kg	Weight lb	Height cm	Height in.	Energy Needs MJ	Energy Needs kcal	Range (kcal)
Infants							
0.0–0.5 yr	6	13	60	24	kg × 0.48	kg × 115	95–145
0.5–1.0 yr	9	20	71	28	kg × 0.44	kg × 105	80–135
Children							
1- yr	13	29	90	35	5.5	1300	900–1800
4–6	20	44	112	44	7.1	1700	1300–2300
7–10 yr	28	62	132	52	10.1	2400	1650–3300
Males							
11–14 yr	45	99	157	62	11.3	2700	2000–3700
15–18 yr	66	145	176	69	11.8	2800	2100–3900
19–22 yr	70	154	177	70	12.2	2900	2500–3300
23–50 yr	70	154	178	70	11.3	2700	2300–3100
51–75 yr	70	154	178	70	10.1	2400	2000–2800
76 + yr	70	154	178	70	8.6	2050	1650–2450
Females							
11–14 yr	46	101	157	62	9.2	2200	1500–3000
15–18 yr	55	120	163	64	8.8	2100	1200–3000
19–22 yr	55	120	163	64	8.8	2100	1700–2500
23–50 y r	55	120	163	64	8.4	2000	1600–2400
51–75 yr	55	120	163	64	7.6	1800	1400–2200
76 + yr	55	120	163	64	6.7	1600	1200–2000
Pregnancy						+300	
Lactation						+500	

[a] From Recommended Dietary Allowances, Revised 1980, Food and Nutrition Board, National Academy of Sciences—National Research Council, Washington, D.C. The data in this table have been assembled from the observed median heights and weights of children, together with desirable weights for adults for mean heights of men (70 in.) and women (64 in.) between the ages of 18 and 34 years as surveyed in the United States population (DHEW/NCHS data).

Energy allowances for the young adults are for men and women doing light work. The allowances for the two older age groups represent mean energy needs over these age spans, allowing for a 2% decrease in basal (resting) metabolic rate per decade and a reduction in activity of 200 kcal/day for men and women between 51 and 75 years; 500 kcal for men over 75 years; and 400 kcal for women over 75. The customary range of daily energy output is shown for adults in the range column and is based on a variation in energy needs of ±400 kcal at any one age, emphasizing the wide range of energy intakes appropriate for any group of people.

Energy allowances for children through age eighteen are based on median energy intakes of children of these ages followed in longitudinal growth studies. Ranges are the 10th and 90th percentiles of energy intake, to indicate range of energy consumption among children of these ages.

picture, I would recommend that short-term treatment (3 to 6 months) be used—again, not because I am convinced of its efficacy but because the potential benefits far outweigh the risks.

Certain diseases associated with the gastrointestinal tract are more common in the elderly—especially in our more affluent societies. Diverticulitis, gall bladder disease, and cancer of the colon are among these diseases. There is evidence which suggests that all three of these may be related to the amount of fiber in the diet (see Chapter 11). The data are strongest for diverticulitis. Low fiber intake increases the prevalence of this disease, probably because it results in decreased transit time and subsequent hardening of stools and constipation. Since constipation is a serious problem in many older people, I would suggest an increase in the fiber content of their diet. This is probably best accomplished by increasing their bran intake.

There is much we still must learn about nutrition and aging but there are certain practical things we can do immediately to improve the nutrition of the elderly. These include providing a balanced diet slightly reduced in calories, relatively low in fats, high in fiber, and particularly, rich in iron, vitamin B_{12}, and calcium.

REVISED RECOMMENDED DIETARY ALLOWANCES—1980

Table 1 shows the recommended dietary allowances, 1980, for all nutrients, for which such allowances have been set. Table 2 is the estimated safe and adequate dietary intakes of additional selected vitamins and minerals. Table 3 shows the mean heights and weights and recommended energy intake for all age groups from birth to beyond 75 years of age.

RECOMMENDED READING

Barrows, C. H., Nutrition, Aging, and Geriatric Programs, *Am. J. Clin. Nutr.*, **25**, 829 (1972).

Exton-Smith, A. N., Physiological Aspects of Aging; Relationship to Nutrition, *Am. J. Clin. Nutr.*, **25**, 853 (1972).

Howell, S. C., and M. B. Loeb, *Nutrition and Aging: A Monograph for Practitioners*, Gerontological Society, Washington, D.C., 1970.

Timiras, P. S., *Developmental Physiology and Aging*, Macmillan, New York, 1972.

Watkins, D. M., Ed., Symposium on Nutrition and Aging, *Am. J. Clin. Nutr.*, **25**, 809 (1972); **26**, 1108 (1973).

Winick, M., Ed., *Nutrition and Aging*, Wiley, New York, 1976.

PART II
NUTRIENT DEFICIENCIES

5

CALORIC DEPRIVATION
IN ADULTS

Although in general excess ingestion of some nutrients, such as calories and saturated fats, presents a greater health problem in America than nutrient deficiencies, the latter still constitute a significant problem to the practicing physician. Primary deficiencies, perhaps with the exception of iron, are rare. However, secondary deficiencies occur quite commonly and must be dealt with in both office and hospital practice. For example, although we see little in the way of primary caloric deprivation or semi-starvation, except in the obese patient trying to reduce, secondary semi-starvation is frequently encountered in the patient with cancer cachexia or the cachexia of other chronic diseases, the patient with anorexia nervosa, and the hospitalized patient who for one reason or another can take little by mouth. Protein deficiency is most common in young children in developing countries but it is still seen in American children, especially among the disadvantaged. Although it is still quite rare, essential fatty acid deficiency is becoming much more common as parenteral nutrition is being continued for longer and longer periods. Even though most of the primary vitamin deficiency diseases have been well controlled, deficiencies of water-soluble vitamins secondary to alcoholism, gastric surgery, or the use of contraceptive pills are quite common. In addition, primary deficiencies of certain fat-soluble vitamins, of various minerals, such as iron, zinc, and perhaps calcium, and of dietary fiber, are being recognized as a major contributor to a number of common chronic illnesses. Thus the pathophysiology and management of the various deficiency states are important to all physicians regardless of their specialty.

CALORIC DEFICIENCY SEMISTARVATION

The body, when deprived of calories for whatever reason, undergoes a series of changes that can be divided into three major stages: (1) depletion of reserves, (2) metabolic adaptation, (3) deterioration and ultimate death.

Depletion of Reserves

The earliest changes, that occur during semistarvation are a loss of body water, which is manifested by polyuria and rapid weight loss, depletion of the glycogen stored in the liver, and depletion of the fat stored in the adipose depot. The conversion of fat stores to energy is accompanied by progressive weight loss. This phase of semistarvation lasts for a period of time that varies depending on the amount of adipose tissue present before the limitation of caloric intake occurs. In severely obese individuals it may last several months, whereas in lean individuals it may be completed in just a few weeks.

Metabolic Adaptation

This phase begins concomitantly with the onset of semistarvation but continues long after reserves have been exhausted. As caloric restriction continues, the body progressively adapts by altering its metabolism. Body water is lost almost exclusively from the intracellular compartments. There is a relative increase in both extracellular and plasma volume. Muscle tissue begins to break down, releasing amino acids, some of which are converted to glucose in the liver to maintain adequate blood sugar levels and to supply energy especially to the central nervous system. Table 1 lists the major changes that the various body compartments undergo.

As caloric restriction continues the entire metabolism of the body undergoes a series of adaptive changes (Table 2). Basal metabolic rate, temperature, and voluntary activity all decrease. The slowing of circulation

Table 1.   Relative changes in body compartments

1. Decrease in intracellular water
2. Increase in extracellular fluid
3. Increase in plasma volume
4. Reduction in total body fat
5. Reduction in lean body mass

Table 2.   Metabolic adaptation to
semistarvation

1. Reduced basal metabolic rate
2. Subnormal temperature
3. Reduced voluntary activity
4. Bradycardia at rest
5. Relative tachycardia during exercise
6. Reduced arterial blood pressure
7. Reduced venous blood pressure
8. Increased circulation time
9. Reduced vital capacity
10. Reduced respiratory efficiency

is manifested by increased circulation time and bradycardia associated
with reduced arterial and venous pressures. In addition there is a reduction
in vital capacity and over-all respiratory efficiency.

All of these changes result in the conservation of energy and are similar
although not identical to changes in body metabolism that are undergone
by certain mammals during hibernation. The mechanisms responsible for
these changes are not well understood. In addition to the adaptation
which takes place in total body metabolism, there are selective effects on
certain organs. These are listed in Table 3. Although grossly and micro-
scopically the brain appears relatively normal, subtle changes in the function of the brain probably occur. Recently it has been shown that the
serotonin concentration in the brain is directly proportional to the concentration of tryptophan, its amino acid precursor. Tryptophan levels in
brain depend on the levels in the blood, which are controlled by the levels
in the diet. Thus the brain hormone serotonin is directly regulated by
diet, especially the quantity and quality of protein consumed. In semistarvation these levels are low.

Table 3.   Selective organ effects of semistarvation

1. Certain organs are almost totally spared: brain, adrenal, skeleton
2. Cell turnover in regenerating organs is impaired: thymus, spleen, bone marrow,
   gastrointestinal mucosa
3. Synthesis of certain proteins in liver is reduced: albumin, lipoprotein
4. Secretion of certain hormones is increased: growth hormone, adrenal hormones

When fully adapted, then, the individual on an extremely low caloric intake will show reduced activity, preferring to stay in bed. Metabolic rate even at rest will be reduced and body temperature is low. Cardiac output is reduced as are both arterial and venous pressure. These reductions, accompanied by the increased plasma volume, lead to a prolongation in the circulation time. The patient, then, is in a precarious circulatory state—in incipient cardiac failure. The selective reduction of liver protein synthesis leads to a fall in plasma albumin concentration and an inability to mobilize lipids from the liver into the general circulation. The reduced regenerative capacity of the gastrointestinal tract will lead to reduced activity of certain gastrointestinal enzymes, which in turn may lead to malabsorption and diarrhea. The increases in adrenal cortical hormone and pituitary growth hormone allow for better mobilization of amino acids and promote gluconeogenesis.

Thus although the individual has "adapted" to the reduced intake of calories, if the reduction is severe enough or prolonged enough a number of distinctly pathological consequences will ensue (Table 4).

The polyuria which has been previously mentioned is accompanied by extreme thirst so that both intake and output of water are markedly increased. The increased extracellular fluid when coupled with the low serum albumin may lead to the appearance of frank edema—the so-called "hunger edema." The lack of regeneration of intestinal cells, the lowered activity of intestinal enzymes, and the edema of the intestinal wall all lead to profound diarrhea, which increases the caloric deficit and may result in water and electrolyte disturbances. Secondary invasion of the injured gut wall by normal gastrointestinal flora may finally occur. Blood sugar levels are often low, especially in the morning after a prolonged fast, and hypoglycemic symptoms may occur. The reduced synthesis of β-lipoprotein by the liver may result in an inability to transport fatty acids from the liver and their subsequent deposition into the liver parenchyma. The low body temperature, even in

Table 4. Pathological consequences of
the adaptive response

1. Polyuria
2. Edema
3. Diarrhea
4. Hypoglycemia
5. Fatty liver
6. Feeling of extreme cold
7. Hypocalcemia and hypokalemia

the face of a lowered basal metabolic rate, often leaves the patient feeling very cold. In addition, the poor circulation may result in cold cyanotic extremities. Finally, the shifts in body fluids, polyuria, and diarrhea may all contribute to low total body potassium, which may be reflected by low serum potassium levels. These same factors, plus the low intake of calcium, may result in hypocalcemia and occasionally in symptoms of tetany.

Thus as semistarvation progresses we have a patient "adapted" to a lower nutrient intake but in a precarious state and often manifesting disturbing symptoms. The adaptive response may break down at any time and the patient will begin to deteriorate rapidly. If therapy is not instituted quickly, death occurs within a short time. As this final stage approaches, the patient begins to manifest certain characteristics (Table 5).

The emaciation becomes profound, the edema if present disappears, the diarrhea worsens, breathing becomes labored, and the patient may die from sudden circulatory collapse, intractable cardiac failure, hypoglycemic coma, or hypokalemia or other electrolyte disturbances. Often the terminal event is widespread infection, which is rapidly fatal under these conditions.

THERAPY

The best approach to this problem is prevention. This is often difficult if the patient's primary disease leads relentlessly to progressive cachexia, such as occurs with certain cancers. It is important to initiate nutritional therapy early in the course of the disease and not to wait until the actual cachexia ensues. High caloric feedings should be instituted and a variety of foods should be available, especially if the patient is anorectic. There is

Table 5. Clinical characteristics of deterioration in semistarvation

1. Large appearing calvarium due to atrophy of facial muscles
2. Bowed head due to weakness of neck muscles
3. Absence of edema (disappears when previously present)
4. Prominence of bony pelvis
5. Flexion of thighs and knees
6. Decreased locomotion and shuffling gait (when ambulatory)
7. Flexor contractures
8. Dyspnea, even at rest
9. Tremors in extremities
10. Profuse, nonremitting, often bloody diarrhea

no use presenting a carefully constructed high calorie diet if the patient will not eat it. If the patient likes one or two particular foods, feed those foods in quantities high enough to provide as many calories as possible. Protein also can be derived from a number of sources. Again determine what your patient will eat and feed it to him—even if it is mainly ice cream and peanut butter. Obviously under these conditions vitamin and mineral supplements should be used. If oral feedings are refused or the oral route is not available, tube feedings and even parenteral feedings should be begun early, before semistarvation has progressed too far. (The actual use of enteral and parenteral solutions is discussed in Chapter 22.)

If the patient is referred to you already in a semistarved condition, determine which of the three phases he or she is in by careful examination and laboratory tests. Look for the signs and symptoms outlined above which are characteristic for each stage. Once you have determined the stage, appropriate therapy can begin.

Patients in the first stage should be placed on a high caloric diet, which they will tolerate. About 3000 to 3500 cal should be consumed, with a protein content of 10 to 15%. Vitamin and mineral supplementation should be given. The patient's weight and skinfold thickness should be monitored and recorded daily. Patients in the second stage must be carefully assessed clinically. If the circulation is badly impaired and the basal metabolic rate is low, then overloading with intravenous fluids or even the feeding of very high caloric diets may precipitate cardiac failure. In the experiments conducted by Keys and co-workers in the early 1950s with volunteers, the most dangerous period was during the early phase of rehabilitation. Several of the patients were thrown into heart failure simply on being fed a high calorie diet—probably because the metabolic rate increased before the blood volume decreased and an already weakened heart could not handle the additional demand under these conditions. For the same reason intravenous therapy must be used carefully and under extremely controlled conditions. Drips should be carefully monitored and run as slowly as possible. Signs of cardiac failure should be looked for and therapy discontinued if they occur. The intravenous route, however, may be the only route open, especially if the patient has severe diarrhea, which is aggravated by oral feedings. Both glucose and amino acids can and should be given under these conditions. Once the patient can tolerate them, oral or tube feedings should be started. Strict attention must be paid to correcting electrolyte imbalances and both calcium and potassium should be supplied. The major principle to remember is not to be overly eager at this stage of therapy. Gradually increasing the nutrient intake is all that is necessary as long as the patient is improving and gaining weight.

It should take a week or perhaps even two weeks before a complete high calorie diet can be consumed. At this point the patient may take 4000 to 4500 cal daily. This is permissible and usually the patient will seek his proper level in a few weeks.

If deterioration has already set in when the patient is first seen, prompt and sometimes "heroic" therapy may be necessary. The circulation may have to be supported as in any patient in shock. Both hypoglycemia and certain electrolyte disturbances may have to be rapidly corrected. Once these emergency measures are taken and the patient is stabilized, nutritional therapy can begin as outlined above.

The prognosis, of course, depends to a great extent on the primary disease. However, if adequate nutrition can be maintained or attained, treatment of the primary disease may be more successful.

Anorexia Nervosa

Anorexia nervosa is the disease seen most often in the United States which perhaps most closely resembles primary semistarvation or caloric restriction. It occurs mainly in adolescent girls shortly after the onset of puberty. The cardinal sign is rapid weight loss in an individual who was previously growing normally. In girls puberty is delayed or reversed and amenorrhea occurs. Some growth in height may continue despite weight loss for a year or more. This weight loss is the result of self-imposed rigorous dieting, which continues even though the patient is hungry. Some patients will consume large meals and then promptly induce vomiting; others may take laxatives or diuretics to exaggerate the weight loss.

There are two theories about the etiology of the disease. One holds that the primary problem is psychologic—disturbed family relationships leading to a child who never develops a sense of autonomy and effectiveness. The other holds that hypothalamic maturation is either retarded or altered, resulting in both the retarded pubertal development and the bizzare feeding behavior.

Whatever the cause, the patient is usually far more emaciated than other physical findings would justify. The signs are primarily those of starvation: pallor, dry skin, lanugo, cold cyanotic extremities, hypothermia, cold intolerance, bradycardia, hypotension, reduced basal metabolic rate, diminished sweating, and amenorrhea in females. In those patients with induced vomiting, tooth erosion may take place. In those taking laxatives or diuretics electrolyte disturbances may be present. Although the patient may be hyperactive in the initial stages, this soon gives way to weakness, apathy, and depression.

Thus the body undergoes an adaptive response identical to the one described above in patients suffering from primary caloric restriction. There is no specific laboratory test diagnostic of anorexia nervosa. The diagnosis is suspected on the basis of history and physical examination and confirmed by ruling out other causes of secondary caloric deprivation.

Treatment is based on the following principles:

1. Educational discussion of the illness.
2. Setting realistic goals.
3. Treatment for malnutrition.
4. Treatment of the emotional disorder.

Although psychotherapy alone may be sufficient in cases where malnutrition is mild, once caloric deprivation has become severe and malnutrition advanced it becomes a life-threatening condition and must be dealt with directly. Correction of the malnutrition is only the first step and must be followed by psychotherapy.

If the patient is consuming too little by mouth to prevent slow starvation and if malnutrition is very severe then tube feedings or intravenous therapy, preferably with amino acids and lipid, should be started. However, I must emphasize again that great care must be taken not to overload an already increased blood volume in a patient who must be considered in incipient heart failure. If oral feedings are possible, by all means use this route, but again with great care. The patient has adapted to caloric restriction and too rapid consumption of calories may increase metabolic rate before adequate circulatory adjustment takes place. The result again could be cardiac failure. A good rule of thumb is to calculate the patient's basal requirements based on her actual basal metabolic rate and her present weight, height, and age. Begin with this and then gradually increase to the requirements at ideal weight. Remember that as along as you can gradually increase caloric intake there is usually no need to hurry.

Thus, depending on the degree of inanition, you might begin with about 1000 to 1250 cal, using the oral route as much as possible but supplementing intravenously if necessary. Gradually, over a period of weeks, you might then increase to 2200 to 2600 cal, depending on the patient's ideal weight.

In patients with anorexia nervosa this plan is often easier to recommend than to carry out. It is important for the physician not to lose patience. Even if it takes months to restore caloric intake, persistence usually pays off, and although the ultimate prognosis must remain guarded and depends to a large extent on the success of psychotherapy, the outlook from a nutritional standpoint is good.

Cancer Cachexia

The cachexia seen in patients with cancer appears to be induced by a combination of events and hence although it is clinically very similar to primary caloric restriction there are very significant differences. Patients with cancer suffer anorexia to various degrees. Although it usually appears after the cancer is well established, it may be an early symptom. The cause of this anorexia is unknown. One component of the cancer cachexia syndrome is a moderate to marked decrease in food intake. There is evidence, however, that utilization of nutrients may be diverted to the tumor from the rest of the body. Thus even with a normal food intake and positive nitrogen balance, cachexia can develop.

The patient with cancer cachexia fails to undergo the complete adaptive response which takes place with primary caloric restriction. Blood pressure, pulse rate, and temperature remain normal, and basal metabolic rate is often elevated rather than decreased. Hence the danger of aggressively feeding a patient with cancer cachexia is much less than with a patient equally emaciated from primary caloric restriction.

Perhaps the main reason for an aggressive approach is that the better the nutritional status of the patient the better the patient will be able to tolerate various kinds of therapy. Higher doses of chemotherapy and radiotherapy can be tolerated in well-nourished patients. Hence, it becomes extremely important to maintain adequate nutrition in a patient being treated for cancer.

Oral feeding is always the preferred route when possible. If anorexia is present, it may preclude voluntary ingestion of an adequate nutrient supply. However even here, certain therapeutic principles may increase voluntary intake. Taste studies in patients with cancer cachexia have shown that they prefer certain foods to others. For example, chicken and fish may be much better tolerated than other meats. Sweet foods are often poorly tolerated. Careful attention to what the patient prefers might reduce the necessity of taking more drastic action.

If oral feeding is not sufficient then tube feeding may be necessary. Here a high calorie, high protein mixture should be employed (see Chapter 22). This can be given several times a day or by nasogastric drip, depending on the patient's tolerance.

Recently intravenous feeding through both peripheral and central veins has become available. This type of parenteral nutrition has become a valuable adjunct in the management of cancer cachexia. Mixtures of sugar, amino acids, and lipid can be given in this manner (see Chapter 22 for details).

Patients with cancer cachexia may become depleted of certain vitamins and minerals. It is important to determine the vitamin and mineral status of such patients and to give supplements when necessary.

SUMMARY

Primary caloric restriction, for whatever reason, will result in a series of changes within the body in which reserves are depleted, adaptation occurs, and if the restriction is prolonged, deterioration and death ensue. The physician makes use of the first stage to induce weight loss in obese patients. However, the adaptive phase, when full blown, although it protects the patient by conserving energy, will result in certain pathologic symptoms. These, in turn, may progress to the point of causing the patient's death even though adaptation has occurred. The entire process must be understood if rational and safe therapy is to be undertaken. Too aggressive a therapeutic approach may result in a reversal of adaptation before the body can tolerate it, which may cause rapid decompensation and even death.

Secondary caloric restriction, as in cancer, results in a clinical picture very similar to primary restriction. However, adequate adaptation does not occur and for this reason deterioration and death are much more rapid. The therapeutic approach here involves supplying excessive amounts of nutrients to overcome the increased utilization of the cancer tissue. The cautious approach taken in treating primary restriction can be supplanted by a much more aggressive approach.

RECOMMENDED READING

Bruch, H., *Eating Disorders: Obesity, Anorexia Nervosa, and the Person Within,* Basic Books, New York, 1973.

Dally, P., *Anorexia Nervosa,* Grune and Stratton, New York, 1969.

Keys, A., G. Brozek, A. Henschel, O. Mickelsen, and H. Taylor, *The Biology of Human Starvation,* University of Minnesota Press, Minneapolis, 1950.

Winick, M., Ed., *Nutrition and Cancer,* Wiley, New York, 1977, pp. 675-695.

Winick, M., Ed., *Hunger Disease,* Wiley, New York, 1979.

6

PROTEIN-CALORIE
DEPRIVATION
IN CHILDREN

All of the metabolic changes that take place in adults as a result of semi-starvation (which were discussed in Chapter 5) occur also in children. However, since children manifest other changes in addition to those seen in adults and since semistarvation, which is often called protein-calorie malnutrition, is more common in children, this chapter will deal with this disease as it occurs in the young child. Again both primary under-nutrition and secondary undernutrition may occur. The former is ex-tremely common in developing countries and in the poorer segments of developed countries. In certain countries as many as 50% of the children are suffering from protein-calorie deficiency. It is estimated that more than 300 million people alive today have suffered from this disease in their childhood years. As we shall see, many may be suffering from its permanent sequelae. Without question, statistically, protein-calorie malnutrition (PCM) is the single greatest health hazard to children in the world. Secondary protein-calorie malnutrition may occur in all societies and in all economic and social classes. In more affluent groups it is much more prevalent that the primary type. Such diseases as cystic fibrosis, pyloric stenosis, infantile gastroenteritis, neoplasm, and other chronic diseases will lead to severe protein-calorie malnutrition. In addition, there is today a growing trend to feed children, even young infants, special types of diets that for adults may be considered fad diets but for infants may result in primary protein-calorie malnutrition or severe undernutrition of certain specific nutrients.

As we have seen, marked reduction in calories and protein in the adult results in depletion of reserves, adaptation, and rapid deterioration. In addition, two types of severe undernutrition have been described in adults, depending on whether edema is present: so-called dry cachexia, and hunger edema. In children, the total depletion of reserves occurs very rapidly because of severely limited fat stores to begin with. Adaptation will begin almost immediately and will take a different form from that in the adult. In addition, the edematous and dry forms constitute more distinct syndromes than in the adult, although gradations between the two exist. Thus we can describe two distinct types of malnutrition in children. The first is infantile marasmus, which characteristically occurs in the infant below 18 months who is not breast fed and cannot be properly bottle fed. This is the type seen in children with cystic fibrosis, pyloric stenosis, or infantile gastroenteritis. The second is kwashiorkor ("disease of the displaced child"), which characteristically occurs in the child over 1 year who is abruptly weaned to a diet low in both calories and protein but relatively lower in protein.

In both of these forms, and in all of the gradations between them, protein-calorie malnutrition results in a characteristic form of adaptation, unique to the young child. The process of growth is severely curtailed—often completely stopped. During the past decade a great deal of research has gone into an attempt to explain this growth-retarding effect. To preserve essential cell functions, the rate of cell division in all organs where it is still occurring is markedly curtailed. In addition, the normal increase in the size of already existing cells does not take place. Thus, one way in which the organs of the body adapt to PCM is by failing to increase either the number or the size of cells. When cell number is reduced the effect is permanent unless rehabilitation is begun during the time that cells are still dividing. By contrast, cell size will reach normal if adequate rehabilitation is accomplished at any time. Thus PCM of early childhood (when cells in the various organs are still rapidly dividing) will result in permanent stunting of growth. Let us now examine the characteristics of the two major types of protein-calorie malnutrition.

Marasmus

Marasmus usually occurs during the first year of life. The primary form of the disease begins when the mother cannot or decides not to breast feed. It is therefore more common in an urban than in a rural setting, where the pressures of city life and the kinds of employment opportunities available work against breast feeding. Bottle feeding under urban slum conditions is usually unsatisfactory. There is no refrigeration, water is often contaminated, sterilization equipment is unavailable, and formula is very expensive and therefore overdiluted. The result is profuse, unremitting diarrhea. The parent often responds by further diluting the formula or switching to a mixture of starch and water which provides a poorer culture medium. The result is semistarvation or protein-calorie malnutrition.

Secondary marasmus may develop when nutrients are not absorbed, as in cystic fibrosis or celiac disease; when nutrients cannot be orally ingested, as in pyloric stenosis or atresia of a portion of the gastrointestinal tract; or in small premature infants who cannot tolerate sufficient intake by mouth. In addition, certain chronic diseases, such as neoplasms or congenital heart disease, may result in growth failure and a cachectic appearance which resembles marasmus.

The child with marasmus is small and underweight and appears generally emaciated. The head may appear enlarged, although this depends to some extent on the age of the child. Both apathy and hyperirritability are present, the infant often lying quietly in bed almost totally unreactive but becoming extremely hyperactive when touched and moved. In most cases there is profuse diarrhea, which often leads to electrolyte imbalance, the most pronounced being hypokalemia. Figure 1 is a picture of a severely marasmic infant. The marasmic infant has exhausted his reserves. There is no liver glycogen, the subcutaneous and even the deep fat is gone, and the muscles are severely atrophic. The diagnosis is established by history, physical examination, and careful anthropometric measurements. These should include length, weight, head circumference, midarm circumference, and subscapular and triceps skinfold measurements, all of which are reduced. The weight:height ratio is usually reduced, especially in the most severe cases. Laboratory studies are of little use in marasmus itself but are important in establishing the primary diagnosis and in documenting and monitoring any electrolyte disturbances which often accompany this condition.

Treatment consists of first correcting the dehydration and electrolyte disturbances with appropriate intravenous therapy. The second step is to begin alimentation, using the simplest form of nutrients available—amino acids or protein hydrolysate and simple sugars, preferably monosaccharides. Alimentation should be undertaken orally, if possible, either in small frequent feedings or by constant nasogastric drip. If even this is not tolerated, the intravenous route may have to be used. Only after this initial period is over (usually a few days but sometimes longer) should regular feedings be attempted. These also must be approached with great care. Intestinal enzyme activity, especially lactase activity, is often diminished. This may result in milk intolerance which could precipitate another serious bout of diarrhea. Hence resumption of milk must be gradual. Dilute feedings should be started. Glucose can be added to increase the caloric

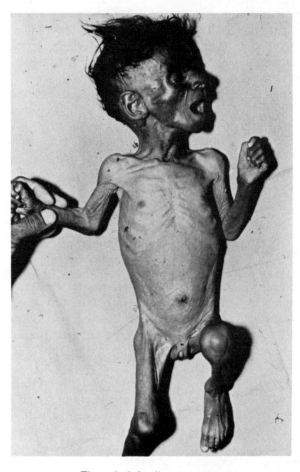

Figure 1. Infantile marasmus.

content. Gradually the concentration can be increased in accordance with the infant's tolerance. Subsequent care involves reinstating breast feeding, if the mother is still lactating and if this is feasible. If not, formula feeding must be used. Formula feeding requires careful instruction to the mother or the same conditions that initiated the problem will recur. If the marasmus is secondary to another disease, the primary cause must be discovered. Measures must be taken to prevent protein-calorie malnutrition from recurring. Sometimes cure of the primary disease is possible (e.g., pyloric stenosis or gastrointestinal atresia) and this will result in the cure also of the conditions leading to marasmus. If the primary disease is chronic (e.g., cystic fibrosis), a diet will have to be established which will prevent marasmus from recurring. Chapter 18 will deal specifically with dietary management of cystic fibrosis and other malabsorptive states. The prognosis of marasmus is always guarded. In severe cases as many as 20% may die even in the best hands. Long-term prognosis in those who recover must also remain guarded because of the possibility of permanent mental sequelae under certain conditions.

Kwashiorkor

Kwashiorkor is almost always a result of primary malnutrition and occurs at the time of weaning when the infant is placed on a diet low in both calories and protein, but relatively lower in protein. It is characterized by edema, skin rash, depigmentation of hair, and hypoalbuminemia in addition to the growth failure previously mentioned. Figure 2 is a typical child suffering from kwashiorkor. The disease may begin insidiously with the

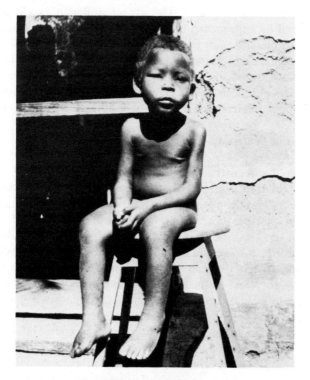

Figure 2. Kwashiorkor

child growing poorly, the appearance of a moon face, gradually increasing edema often beginning around the eyes, and then the appearance of the rash and hair changes. However, frank kwashiorkor often is precipitated acutely by the occurrence of infection, such as measles, in a chronically malnourished child. Because of the edema, the weight loss may not be apparent, but height will be decreased. Head circumference may be reduced, though less than in marasmus. The edema is pitting in nature and effusions into body cavities are rare, in contrast to the adult form of hunger edema. In contrast to marasmus, a number of laboratory findings are markedly abnormal. Serum albumin is always low and when it drops to 2.5 mg/cc or below frank edema appears. Serum levels of lipoprotein are low, resulting in an inability to transport lipids from the liver and finally in fatty deposition in the liver itself. The child with kwashiorkor will often have diarrhea, although this is not as universal as with marasmus.

Treatment follows the same principles as for marasmus, except that the intravenous fluids must be used with even greater care to prevent circulatory overload. The introduction of high protein foods should begin as soon as possible and should be gradual to avoid intolerances due to inactivity of intestinal enzymes. The use of milk, an excellent source of protein, should be approached in the same way as in the marasmic infant. Diuresis, often massive, may begin at almost any time during early therapy. During this period careful attention should be given to the child's electrolyte state. Potassium and magnesium supplementation is often necessary during this phase. The prognosis must remain guarded both from the standpoint of initial recovery and from the standpoint of ultimate mental development.

Milder Forms of Protein-Calorie Malnutrition

All gradations between the two distinct types of PCM occur in children. Some of the children will show signs of marasmus but they may be hypo-albuminemic and mildly edematous. Others may have signs of kwashiorkor superimposed on the emaciation and muscular atrophy of marasmus. However, the majority of children suffering from PCM exhibit evidence of growth failure, low weight for height, reduced midarm circumference, and reduction in the thickness of the skinfolds. The diagnosis is made entirely on history and anthropometry. Treatment consists of instituting a diet adequate in both protein and calories. Prognosis is good but long-term mental development may be impaired under certain conditions.

Thus, reduced intake of calories and protein in young infants, either in its primary form or secondary to some other disease, may result in one of two distinct syndromes (marasmus or kwashiorkor), a combination of the two, or, in its milder form, in growth failure alone. Recently we have been seeing cases of all of these appear as a result of fad dieting applied to infants, especially at the time of weaning. Physicians must remain alert to the signs and symptoms of PCM since it is one disease that is preventable, usually curable, and unfortunately extremely common.

EARLY MALNUTRITION AND MENTAL DEVELOPMENT

In the early 1960s data began to accumulate from a number of sources which suggested that severe early malnutrition might permanently alter brain structure as well as impair brain function. Both of these conclusions were based on animal experiments and studies of human populations.

Animal Studies

In animals, malnutrition during the nursing period and even in utero was shown to reduce brain weight, retard the rate of brain cell division, impair the process of myelination, and reduce the number of dendritic arborizations. In addition, secretion of such neural hormones as serotonin, norepinephrine and acetylcholine was altered. These changes were found to be permanent if the malnutrition occurred during the time when these processes were progressing at their most rapid rate.

Animals malnourished by identical means and for identical periods of time showed a series of behavioral changes some of which persisted throughout their lives. Such animals were unable to negotiate mazes properly, had difficulty in extinguishing previously conditioned responses, and could not "learn" certain problems. The initial conclusion was that these animals had an impaired learning ability which persisted throughout life. The implications, of course, were staggering. More careful interpretation of the data made it clear that such a depressing conclusion was not warranted, since the motivation to perform, which was used as a measure of learning, was often a food reward and previously restricted animals might very well respond differently to such a reward than animals that had never been exposed to food restriction. Hence a different type of experiment was devised. Animals who had previously been malnourished were compared to control animals in an open field. They were merely placed in a box with four squares on the floor and the number of times they traversed the squares was counted. In addition, the level of excitement of these animals was measured by counting the number of times they reared on their hind legs and the number of urinations and defecations. Results of a series of these experiments demonstrated that the previously malnourished animals had decreased exploratory behavior and were more excitable than animals reared in the normal manner. There was no question that behavioral changes occurred and that these changes were permanent. What the changes actually meant, however, was unclear. What also soon became unclear was to what extent these behavioral changes were due to early malnutrition and to what extent they were due to the rest of the animals' early environment. These animals were malnourished while nursing and although a variety of techniques were used—either increasing nursing litter size, restricting maternal diet, or surgically removing some of the teats—in every case the maternal–pup interaction was severely altered. Was it these alterations or the actual malnutrition that was producing these behavioral effects? A number of observations suggested that both might be contributing factors. Simple isolation of the pup from the mother for periods of time even if the nutrition was adequate resulted in behavioral changes similar to those just described. By contrast, stimulating animals in a variety of ways at the same time as they were being undernourished reduced and sometimes obliterated the behavioral deficit. These studies led to a hypothesis that malnutrition early in life exerted its primary effects by functionally isolating the animal from its environment and thereby blocking the necessary stimuli from reaching the developing animal at a critical time in its life. A ray of hope was injected into what had previously been a very dark picture. Perhaps the effects of such early malnutrition could be reversed if the animal were subsequently reared in an environment where extra stimulation was provided. Experiments which followed quickly demonstrated that many of the expected behavioral deficits could be avoided and some could even be reversed. Obviously extrapolation to humans could not be made from these data. However, simultaneously with these animal experiments a number of human studies were being conducted and were suggesting a similar story.

Human Studies

The early human studies, like the early animal studies, tried to examine the effects of severe malnutrition in infancy on subsequent learning. Usually, IQ tests were used to measure outcome. At first, such tests had to be standardized for the culture in which they were being used. Even after this was done it was evident that children previously malnourished in early life performed poorly on these tests. What did this mean? Were these tests a valid indication of how well children would do in their own culture? This certainly was not known and in fact is not known today. A much more serious problem in interpreting the results had to do with the difficulty of isolating malnutrition from the rest of the complex cultural and socioeconomic environment within which the infant was reared—essentially the same problem encountered in the animal experiments but much more difficult to deal with in human populations. A series of studies were devised in an attempt to isolate nutrition from the other possible variables. One particularly innovative approach was carried out in Jamaica. Children who were admitted to the hospital severely malnourished and who subsequently recovered were compared with their siblings and with a control child who had never previously been malnourished but who came from the same general socioeconomic background. The results showed that years later the index cases had the lowest IQ and school performance, the siblings were intermediate, and the control children did best. In addition to IQ and performance other behavioral parameters were measured and again they indicated that the previously malnourished child showed the most abnormalities. Thus the data suggested that malnutrition in addition to the other environmental factors contributed to the subsequent poorer development of these children but that the poor environment itself (as demonstrated in the siblings) also was contributing to faulty development. In the early 1970s two studies, one with children with cystic fibrosis and the second with children with pyloric stenosis, were reported. All of these children were severely malnourished early in life. However, all were from middle class American homes, an environment quite different from the environment which results in primary malnutrition. The results showed that by 5 years of age, these children had normal IQs. These data were interpreted to demonstrate that the expected effects of malnutrition could be prevented if the rest of the environment were normal. Could subsequent enrichment of the environment prevent the effects of early primary malnutrition on subsequent development? Two recent studies suggest that the answer is yes. Korean orphans malnourished during the first year of life and adopted before age 3 by American families were compared with moderately nourished and well-nourished Korean children similarly adopted. Results demonstrated that the most malnourished group of children had IQ and achievement scores at or slightly above United States norms. The other two groups did even better. Figure 3 summarizes the results. A second study in American black children compared multiple foster home care with single foster home care. The data demonstrate that previously malnourished children (determined by reduced stature) if placed in a single stable foster home did as well as well-nourished children in the same environment. By contrast, malnourished children who are exposed to multiple placements do neither as well as well-nourished children under the same conditions nor as well as malnourished children in the stable environment. These data strongly suggest that early nutrition and the

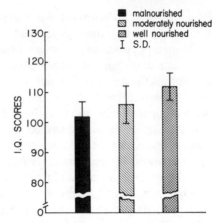

Figure 3. Current IQ scores of previously malnourished, moderately nourished, and well nourished Korean orphans who were adopted by American families prior to age 3.

rest of the socioeconomic environment interact in determining subsequent development. In addition, they suggest that even children who suffered from primary malnutrition and were reared in a deprived environment can develop normally if they are subsequently reared in a stable or enriched environment. How early must this environment enrichment take place? We have not yet been able to establish this timing. A very recent study similar to the first one with Korean orphans, but examining children adopted after age 3 suggests that all of the children, regardless of previous nutrition, are doing worse than those in the former study. The previously malnourished children are doing least well and are performing below United States norms. However, their performance is still better than one would expect if they had been returned to their original environment (Figure 4).

How can we translate these data into practical programs? What kind of environmental enrichment is necessary to reverse the developmental consequences of poor nutrition and poor environment early in life? Are early head start programs or day care programs the proper approach? In spite of these unanswered questions, we have learned a great deal in the past two decades. We have in fact come full cycle—from considering the brain damage and mental retardation irreversible to seeing the situation as not only preventable but potentially reversible. Here, as in many areas of biomedical science, prevention and reversal of the disease process may precede our full understanding of the mechanisms by which the abnormality occurs.

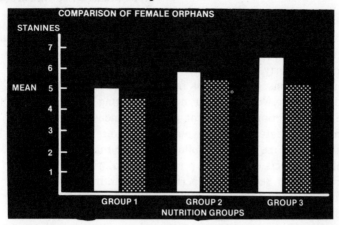

Figure 4. Comparisons of Korean orphans adopted before age 3 (solid bars) and after age 3 (stippled bars): Group 1—malnourished, Group 2—moderately nourished, Group 3—well nourished.

Protein-Calorie Deficiency and Infection

A serious problem in patients with primary protein-calorie malnutrition or with protein-calorie malnutrition secondary to some other disease is concomitant infection. The problem of the interaction of infection and undernutrition has two important aspects: (1) infection depletes the nutritional reserves of the host and increases nutritional requirements, both of which aggravate the protein-calorie malnutrition; (2) The incidence of infection is increased in patients with severe protein-calorie malnutrition, and the course of infection is particularly virulent in these patients.

Table 1 outlines some important effects of infection on nutritional status.

Thus in a patient with protein-calorie malnutrition any infection will aggravate the malnutrition by increasing calorie expenditure, wasting nitrogen, and decreasing further caloric intake. In populations where

Table 1.   Effects of infection on nutritional status

Increased nutrient requirement	Infection increases metabolism
	Infection results in negative nitrogen balance
Decreased nutrient intake	Infection often results in anorexia

nutritional status is marginal, such as in some third world countries and some poverty areas in our own country, this increased nutrient requirement and decreased nutrient intake secondary to infection have become part of the ecology of poverty.

Under conditions of marginal nutrition, growth rate may be slightly retarded but otherwise children may be getting along reasonably well. Suddenly an infection occurs, for example, measles; food intake drops, requirements increase, and frank malnutrition often in the form of kwashiorkor ensues. As one infection follows another many children succumb to the combined effects of infection and protein-calorie malnutrition. In those who survive, such sequelae as permanent stunting and retarded mental development may remain.

Not only does infection worsen malnutrition but protein-calorie malnurition "breeds" infection and the course of such infections is often atypical and rapidly progressive. For example, it has been noted many times that during widespread famine, infections often rapidly reach epidemic proportions and decimate the population. Whether this is due to a breakdown in general host resistance is not yet fully understood.

The severity of certain infections increases markedly when the host is in a malnourished state, although often a minimum of the usual symptoms and signs of the particular infection will be present. Patients with measles may show only mild elevations of temperature and no rash and yet will rapidly succumb. Tuberculosis will often progress rapidly, with bone disease, meningitis, and widespread tuberculous pneumonia.

Recent studies suggest a defect in cellular immunity in patients suffering from protein-calorie malnutrition. There is a lack of skin response to certain antigens. For example, in patients with tuberculosis the intradermal tuberculin test is often negative. In animals, skin grafts are not readily rejected. Most of the evidence currently available points to a defect in T-cells. By contrast humoral immunity, as measured by the amount of various globulins produced in response to an antigenic stimulus, is relatively normal. Finally, total white blood count is often reduced and there is a relative lymphocytosis.

In summary, protein-calorie malnutrition increases the severity of infections and many infections usually easily contained by the host spread widely. This is due, at least in part, to an impairment in cellular immunity, the exact nature of which is still under investigation. In addition, infection increases the severity of protein-calorie malnutrition by reducing intake, increasing requirements, and depleting reserves, This vicious cycle of protein-calorie malnutrition and infection is the most common cause of death in developing countries.

RECOMMENDED READING

Manocha, S. L., *Malnutrition and Retarded Human Development,* Thomas, Springfield, Ill., 1972.

McCance, R. A., and E. M. Widdowson, The Determinants of Growth and Form, *Proc. Roy. Soc. Brit.,* **185**, 1 (1974).

Owen, G. M., K. M. Kram, P. J. Garry, J. E. Lowe, and A. H. Lubin, A Study of Nutritional Status of Preschool Children in the United States, 1968–1970, *Pediatrics,* **53**, 4, Part II, Suppl. (1974).

Scrimshaw, N. S., and J. E. Gordon, *Malnutrition, Learning, and Behavior,* MIT Press, Cambridge, Mass., 1968.

Van Duzen, J. P., Protein and Calorie Malnutrition Among Preschool Navajo Indian Children, *Am. J. Clin. Nutr.,* **22**, 1362 (1969).

Winick, M., Ed., *Nutrition and Development,* Wiley, New York, 1972.

Winick, M., *Malnutrition and Brain Development,* Oxford University Press, New York, 1976.

Winick, M., Ed., *Human Nutrition,* Plenum, New York, 1979.

7

ESSENTIAL FATTY ACID DEFICIENCY

For years we have believed that certain fatty acids were essential in the human diet. However, because of the difficulty in inducing complete deficiency and the length of time necessary for symptoms to occur direct evidence was difficult to obtain. Recently, with the advent of total parenteral nutrition carried on for long periods of time without any lipid, definite symptoms of fatty acid deficiency have occurred. Such symptoms can be prevented or reversed by giving intralipid preparations which contain linoleic acid. Thus what was formerly strongly suspected has now become an established fact. Man has an absolute requirement for at least one fatty acid and is unable to compensate for its lack. Prolonged deficiency will lead to symptoms which although nonspecific can be attributed to a lack of this dietary factor. Therefore it is important that the physician in practice, especially one caring for a patient who is receiving total parenteral nutrition, understand the pathogenesis of this disease and that he be able to recognize its symptoms and treat it adequately.

BIOCHEMISTRY OF ESSENTIAL FATTY ACID DEFICIENCY

Figure 1 is an extremely simplified diagram depicting the major biochemical events in the formation of essential fatty acid (EFA) deficiency. Linoleic acid ($C18:2\omega6$) is usually supplied in the diet and serves as the normal precursor of the essential fatty acid for humans, arachidonic acid ($C20:4\omega6$). If EFA deficiency occurs, the concentration of arachidonic acid drops. Oleic acid ($C18:1\omega9$), which can be synthesized by the body and hence

60

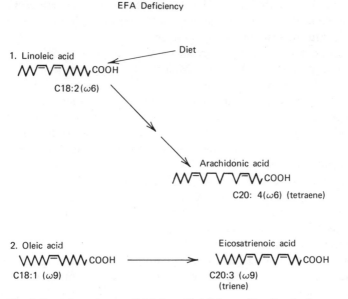

Figure 1. Metabolic pathway in essential fatty acid deficiency. Reaction 1 when present will inhibit reaction 2. In EFA deficiency, reaction 2 is stimulated.

does not need to be supplied in the diet, is converted to eicosatrienoic acid (C20:3ω9) during EFA deficiency. This reaction is normally inhibited by arachidonic acid. Thus the concentration of trienes (acids with three double bonds) increases whereas the concentration of tetraenes (acids with four double bonds) drops. The triene:tetraene ratio increases markedly and this is the cardinal biochemical sign of EFA deficiency both in plasma and in tissues. If you suspect the diagnosis of EFA deficiency a plasma triene:tetraene ratio should be determined. The ratio in plasma is normally 0.4. In EFA deficiency it may rise to 5 or higher.

CLINICAL FEATURES OF ESSENTIAL FATTY ACID DEFICIENCY

Essential Fatty Acid Deficiency in Animals

Essential fatty acid deficiency has been produced in rats by feeding them a totally fat free diet. Such animals exhibit skin and hair abnormalities, necrosis of the tail, poor wound healing, and capillary fragility. Histologically one sees hyperplasia of all three layers of the epidermis, infiltration of the dermis by round cells, hyperkeratosis of hair follicles, and degeneration of hair shafts. Thus one of the characteristic findings in experimental EFA deficiency, similar to what is found in the human disease, is changes in the skin and its appendages.

Young animals made deficient in EFA fail to grow. Adult animals show impaired reproductive capacities. Males exhibit degeneration of the tubular lining in the testes and a cessation of spermatogenesis. Females have irregular estrous cycles, impaired gestation and lactation, fetal resorption, and degeneration of luteal cells. In addition, there is an increased metabolic rate and a reduced resistance to stress in adult animals of both sexes.

At a more fundamental level, increased cell membrane fragility and permeability have been reported. There is mitochondrial swelling, increased mitochondrial oxidation of citric acid cycle intermediates, and a reduced capacity of lysosomes to release certain enzymes. The electrocardiograph shows a notching of the QRS complex, which is specific for EFA deficiency. Some investigators have reported that a deficiency in EFA may lead to a marginal magnesium deficiency. Finally, essential fatty acids are necessary for the formation of certain prostaglandins. It has been postulated that arachidonic acid is essential because it serves as a precursor of prostaglandins.

Essential Fatty Acid Deficiency in Man

In man, the symptoms of EFA deficiency are most prónounced during the perinatal period because requirements are greater during rapid periods of growth and supply is limited during this period. The human infant is born with a limited supply of EFA (linoleic acid comprises only about 1% of newborn adipose tissue) and many infants are fed formulas derived from cow's milk or containing coconut oil, which are very low in EFA content.

Thus in studies where newborn infants were fed skimmed milk formulas (containing only 0.1% of calories as linoleic acid) more than half developed dry scaly skin within 6 weeks. Pathologically there is a disappearance of the stratum corneum, hyperplasia of the epidermis, and shrinkage of the cells resulting in prominent intracellular bridges. Keratinization is impaired and the stratum granulosum is thickened. Finally there is hyperkeratosis of hair follicles, degeneration of hair shafts, and shrinkage of sebaceous glands. Again the cardinal symptoms are changes in the skin and its appendages. These are recognized clinically as dry, flaky, scaly skin which is thick and rough and which is devoid of the fine, thin hair often seen in young infants. In addition to these skin symptoms the infant with EFA deficiency fails to grow, even on a diet that is adequate both in calories and in protein for normal growth. This growth failure is probably due to a less efficient utilization of calories.

In adults the major symptom is a dry, flaky skin rash, which though milder than in children can be extremely troublesome. In adults EFA deficiency is usually seen in patients maintained for a few weeks to several months on total parenteral nutrition without any source of lipid. In both adults and children there is an increased triene:tetraene ratio, which rises sharply after the dietary linoleic acid content falls below 1% of the total caloric intake. This increased ratio is diagnostic of the disease. More precise biochemical studies will demonstrate an actual *decrease* in arachidonic acid and an *increase* in eicosatrienoic acid.

Recent studies have shown that the developing brain, especially during its period of rapid myelination, may be particularly sensitive to EFA deficiency. In rats raised from birth on EFA deficient mothers, brain weight was reduced, as was total lipid concentration of the brain. In addition, the newly deposited myelin had an abnormal fatty acid composition. Finally, the triene:tetraene ratio in whole brain phosphoglycerides and in synaptosomes and myelin was elevated.

In one study puppies were raised from birth either on dextrose and water only or on total parenteral nutrition (TNP) consisting of the same amino acid and dextrose solution usually given to patients. When these animals were compared with animals reared on the mother's milk it was noted that the animals on TPN grew normally whereas those raised on 10% dextrose alone grew very little. There was a rapid and marked increase in serum and brain triene:tetraene ratios in the TPN reared animals, whereas the dextrose and water animals who also received no lipid and hence no EFA had a slower increase. Thus for essential fatty acid deficiency to occur rapidly, normal growth must be occurring.

The functional significance, if any, of the abnormal triene:tetraene ratio in the brains of these animals is unknown. However, rats reared in this manner show reproducible behavioral abnormalities. The data so far available suggest that both the ratio and the behavioral changes can be corrected by feeding linoleic acid.

Preliminary data in human infants who have had to be reared for long periods on TPN demonstrate an abnormally high triene:tetraene ratio in the serum. Moreover, in a few infants who have died and whose brains have been examined, the data suggest that the myelin which was deposited was abnormal.

From what has been described above there is little doubt that EFA deficiency is a real problem in certain patients and a potential problem in many others. How do we as physicians prevent this deficiency in those at high risk and treat it when it presents itself?

As we have noted, the individual at greatest risk is the young growing child. During the first year of life the vast majority of fat in the diet is derived from breast milk, infant formula, or whole cow's milk, depending on the age of the infant and how he is fed. With the emphasis on prevention of coronary artery disease many pediatricians are concerned with the cholesterol content of the diet and are using skimmed milk directly after weaning from breast or infant formula. This should not be done during the first year of life, especially if other sources of fat in the diet, for example, eggs, are being restricted. Partially skimmed milk will probably supply adequate quantities of EFA if polyunsaturated fatty acids are supplied from vegetable oils and fish sources as well. After the first year of life if the diet is varied enough to supply an intake of linoleic acid of 1% or more of calories, skimmed milk can be used. If skimmed milk is used, care should be taken to supply vegetable oil and certain fish sources of linoleic acid.

In adults, EFA deficiency is unlikely to occur unless the diet is extremely restricted in all sources of fat.

In patients receiving total parenteral nutrition, EFA deficiency has become almost inevitable if no lipid is being given. It can be prevented either by supplying small amounts of linoleic acid in the form of vegetable oil by mouth, if possible, or by using intralipid preparations if the oral route is not accessible.

Recent studies in animals and in a few patients on TPN suggest that the skin manifestations of EFA deficiency and the abnormal triene:tetraene ratios in serum and in tissues can be reversed by rubbing olive oil on the skin. Presumably, enough linoleic acid can be absorbed by this route to correct the deficiency. More studies are necessary to confirm these important observations.

In summary, EFA deficiency is a real and potential disease in an increasing number of people. Table 1 summarizes the major clinical and biochemical findings as well as the main approaches to prevention and therapy. Those at risk include young infants, especially those being fed low fat diets, and either children or adults receiving total parenteral nutrition. The main symptoms in children are growth failure and a dry, scaly rash which may be confused with seborrheic dermatitis. There is some concern that young infants who are EFA deficient may be depositing myelin with an abnormal fatty acid content. In adults the skin lesions predominate. In both children and adults the serum triene:tetraene ratio is elevated, and this elevated ratio is diagnostic. Prevention in children involves assuring an adequate supply of linoleic acid, and hence during the first year totally skimmed milk should not be used, especially in an infant whose other sources of fat are being restricted. Later, skimmed milk can be used but care should be taken to supply adequate amounts of polyunsaturated fatty acids from vegetable or fish sources. In adults,

Table 1. Essential Fatty Acid Deficiency

Clinical symptoms	Dry scaly and flaky skin with loss of hair over affected parts—adults and children Growth failure—children Possible abnormal myelin deposition—children
Biochemical findings	Increased triene:tetraene ratio in serum and tissues. Decreased concentration of arachidonic acid and increased concentration of eicosatrienoic acid in serum and tissues
Prevention	Supply 1% or more of total caloric intake as linoleic acid. Major practical step is to discourage totally skimmed milk during the first year of life
Treatment	Oral linoleic acid if possible; if not, use intravenous route. Possibility of using application on skin as a route of administration of EFA is being investigated

unless the individual is consuming a diet which is markedly restricted in all fats, there is little risk of EFA deficiency. However, if an individual is on TPN, then linoleic acid should be supplied either by mouth, intravenously, or, if recent studies are confirmed, by rubbing it on the skin.

RECOMMENDED READING

Essential Fatty Acid Deficiency in Continuous-Drip Alimentation, *Nutr. Rev.*, **33**, 329 (1975).

Goodhart, R. S., and M. E. Shils, *Modern Nutrition in Health and Disease*, 6th ed., Lea and Febiger, Philadelphia, 1980.

Paulsrud, J. R., Essential Fatty Acid Deficiency in Infants Induced by Fat Free Intravenous Feeding, *Am. J. Clin. Nutr.*, **25**, 897 (1972).

8

DEFICIENCIES OF
FAT-SOLUBLE VITAMINS

A vitamin is an essential nutrient because the body is unable to synthesize it from other sources. It is necessary in very small amounts and hence falls into the class of micronutrients. Deficiency will result in symptoms that will ultimately progress to death if the vitamin is not supplied. The vitamins can be divided into two major groups: those which are soluble in water and those which are soluble in fat. This chapter and the next will discuss the manifestations of a deficiency of one or more of these substances.

The fat-soluble vitamins, A, D, K, and E, have certain things in common. Primary deficiency diseases are more frequent and more severe in children than in adults (Table 1), probably because children have lower reserve stores of these vitamins and because requirements are higher during the growing period. Hence deficiencies of vitamins K and E manifest themselves shortly after birth and deficiencies of vitamins A and D usually occur during early childhood. All of the fat-soluble vitamins are stored within the body and therefore reserves can be made available when dietary supply is low. All of the fat-soluble vitamins are carried from the intestines to the liver bound to chylomicrons and all are modified or bound in the liver and then released into the general circulation.

VITAMIN A (RETINOL) DEFICIENCY

Figure 1 is a diagram of how vitamin A is absorbed, metabolized, and utilized by the body. There are two dietary forms of vitamin A. Retinol

66

Table 1. Fat-soluble vitamin deficiency in children and adults

Vitamin	Children	Adults
A	*Night blindness*—aldehyde formed from retinol is an essential component of visual purple, which is essential for stimulating rods in night vision *Xerosis conjunctiva*—Bitot's spots *Xerosis cornea—keratomalacia*—perforation of cornea, prolapse of iris, extrusion of lens, infection of entire eyeball *Growth failure* (present in animals)	*Follicular keratosis, night blindness, xerosis conjunctiva*—rarely progressing to further eye disease
D	*Rickets*—child may appear well nourished even fat and flabby; restless, pale, poor muscle tone, abnormal limb positions, delayed sitting and walking, delayed tooth eruption; craniotabes, enlarged epiphyses, rachitic rosary, bossing of frontal and parietal bones, bowing of extremities	*Osteomalacia*—skeletal pain, muscle weakness, kyphosis, loss of bone density often accompanies osteoporosis in older people
E	*Hemolytic anemia*—in premature infants which may be exaggerated on administration of iron	
K	*Hemorrhagic disease of the newborn*—intracranial hemorrhage	

itself comes from animal sources usually associated with fat; for example, fish liver oils. However, the major source of vitamin A in our diets is β-carotene, which comes from plant sources; for example, carrots or other yellow vegetables. The β-carotene is cleaved at its central double bond and then both ends are converted to retinol in the intestinal mucosa. Retinol, from whatever source, is converted to retinol palmitate again in the intestinal mucosa and in this form it is transported to the liver bound to chylomicrons.

The liver synthesizes a specific protein, retinol-binding protein (RBP), which binds retinol, and it is in this bound complex as well as in a complex with another protein, prealbumin, that vitamin A circulates to the peripheral organs and tissues. Excess vitamin A is stored in the liver as retinol esters. The level of vitamin A in the serum or in the tissues controls the release of

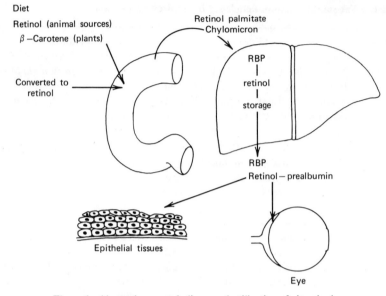

Figure 1. Absorption, metabolism, and utilization of vitamin A.

RBP from the liver and hence the availability of vitamin A. Thus as serum and tissue levels of vitamin A fall, the liver releases more vitamin A complexed to RBP. Conversely, if the serum or tissue levels are high, excess vitamin A is stored in the liver in the form of esters.

Not all of the actions of vitamin A have yet been defined. In fact, the only physiologic function of vitamin A that has been clearly defined on a biochemical basis is its role in vision. Rhodopsin, which is an integral part of the visual purple necessary for night vision, is synthesized, in part, from retinol. Hence in vitamin A deficiency, night vision is impaired and often absent. Beyond its role in the visual cycle vitamin A is known to be required for growth, reproduction, and the maintenance of life. More specifically, it is involved in maintaining the integrity of epithelial tissue, and recent evidence suggests that it is important in the synthesis of glyco-proteins. However, the exact manner in which vitamin A functions in these systems is still not known.

Vitamin A deficiency is a major health problem throughout much of the third world. It is confined mainly to children, although its scars can be seen in many adults. The major manifestations affect the eyes and can be classified in five stages as outlined in Table 2 (from Oomen, 1976).

Night blindness (Stage 1) is due to a functional impairment of the retina and is very difficult to diagnose because the subject is usually a small

Table 2. Classification of eye changes in vitamin A deficiency

Stage 1 Only night blindness present

Stage 2 Xerosis of the conjunctiva, with or without night blindness and with or without Bitot's spots

Stage 3 Xerosis of the cornea; superficial reversible changes of the corneal epithelium

Stage 4 Irreversible corneal changes, involving the corneal stroma leading to loss of substance and perforation, and possibly to keratomalacia

Stage 5 Scars presenting as nebula, a total or partial leucoma, a staphyloma or phthisis bulbi

child (1 to 4 years old). The physician usually must rely on the history given by the mother that the child is unable to see after dusk.

Xerosis of the conjunctiva (Stage 2) is usually the first visual manifestation of xerophthalmia. The conjunctiva appears dry and dull and does not reflect light in its normal shiny manner. Xerosis of the conjunctiva is usually accompanied by night blindness and often by Bitot's spots, an accumulation of debris and fatty material near the limbus of the eye, especially lateral to the cornea (Figure 2).

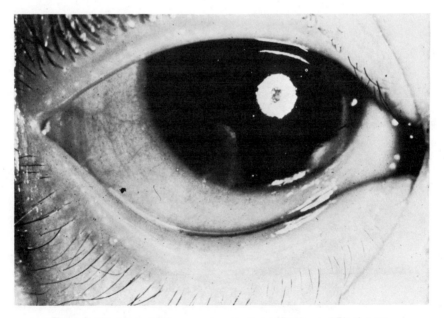

Figure 2. Vitamin A deficiency; early corneal opacification and Bitot's spot.

In the second visual stage (Stage 3) the cornea itself becomes opaque and dry. Soon erosions or small perforations appear. This stage is short and if it is treated quickly with large doses of vitamin A, the changes can be reversed (Figure 3).

Once the deeper layers of the cornea are affected (Stage 4) the damage is irreversible. In the worst cases the cornea "liquefies" and melts away, causing large perforations and extrusion of the iris, the lens, and the vitreous body (Figure 4). If in this stage intraocular pressure can be restored, the result is an ugly bulging staphyloma or a flat whitish leucoma. If pressure is not restored, the eyeball shrinks, leaving only a scarred remnant of the organ.

The scarring effects (Stage 5), therefore, are variable. They do, however, present evidence of xerophthalmia to the experienced observer. In an area endemic for vitamin A deficiency such scars developing in the third or fourth year of life are almost pathognomonic of a previous episode of xerophthalmia.

Vitamin A deficiency is the major cause of blindness in the third world. In India alone it results in hundreds of thousands of blind children annually. In the developed world these severe manifestations of vitamin A deficiency are extremely rare. However milder forms are not infrequently

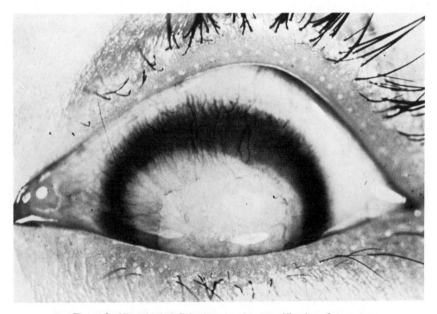

Figure 3. Vitamin A deficiency; complete opacification of cornea.

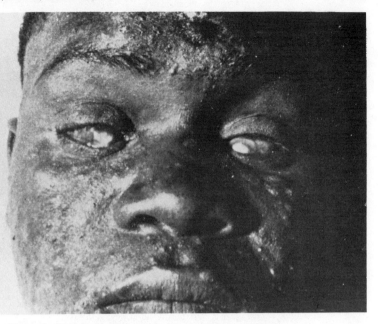

Figure 4. Vitamin A deficiency; terminal scarring and blindness.

encountered. The recent ten state nutrition survey and the young child survey demonstrated low serum levels among certain groups of the lower socioeconomic segments of the population. Some of our dietary "cults" recommend diets which are grossly deficient in vitamin A, and children subjected to such diets have developed overt vitamin A deficiency. Signs may include follicular keratitis (Figure 5) as well as the eye changes. In a patient with serious signs of vitamin A deficiency prevention of blindness requires immediate massive doses of vitamin A.

The prevention of vitamin A deficiency should be approached by dietary means. In countries where the disease is rampant periodic large oral doses have been administered as a public health measure. Since the vitamin can be stored, this approach has met with some success. A regime such as this, in which 60 mg (200,000 IU) of an oily solution of retinol is given by mouth every 3 to 6 months, is currently being used in India, Indonesia, Bangladesh, and elsewhere. This procedure, however, is a passive one and should be replaced as rapidly as possible with the institution of a diet adequate in vitamin A, usually in the form of carotene, from green leafy vegetables of endogenous origin.

In the United States the use of these high doses of vitamin A for prevention of deficiency is contraindicated. This vitamin in high doses is extremely

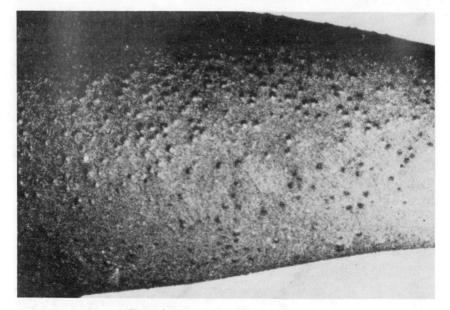

Figure 5. Vitamin A deficiency; skin rash.

toxic (toxicity of vitamins is discussed in Chapter 15) and since serious deficiency is rare such extreme measures should almost never be employed.

Vitamin A is abundant in our food supply and therefore there are almost no indications for supplementation in an otherwise healthy person, even if serum vitamin A levels are low. Increasing the amount of green or yellow vegetables or the consumption of margarine should supply ample amounts. The physician, however, must remain alert to the possibility of this deficiency. If it is suspected, serum vitamin A levels can be obtained. However, since therapy is extremely simple and totally without untoward effects if dietary means are employed, it can be instituted as soon as the suspicion is present. If actual symptoms, such as night blindness, are present, a vitamin A supplement of no more than 40,000 IU can be given daily for a short time until the symptoms disappear. This supplement should be combined with the institution of an adequate diet and discontinued as soon as the patient is eating properly.

VITAMIN D DEFICIENCY

Deficiency of vitamin D, like deficiencies of other fat-soluble vitamins, is most common and most severe in young children. It may occur during the first year of life, and has even been diagnosed in utero by examining X-rays of fetuses of vitamin D-deficient mothers.

During the early part of this century, rickets, the classic vitamin D-deficiency disease, was extremely common in the United States and in Europe. However, with the addition of vitamin D to milk, primary rickets has been almost eliminated in most developed countries. In developing countries, however, vitamin D-deficient rickets remains one of the major cripplers of children.

Early rachitic changes can be detected by X-rays. In a small child the epiphyses of the wrists are splayed and ragged in appearance (Figure 6). As growth progresses and weight-bearing begins, the tibias become soft because of poor calcification and slowly bend (Figure 7). At the costochondral junctions, faulty calcification results in a series of beadlike projections just lateral to the sternum, known as the rachitic rosary (Figure 8). Hence the child with active rickets is short and deformed, and has extremely painful and tender epiphyses.

The disease responds dramatically to small doses of vitamin D and can be prevented by adequate exposure to sunlight or by eating foods containing vitamin D, such as oily fish and enriched foods.

In more advanced countries, secondary rickets—also called vitamin

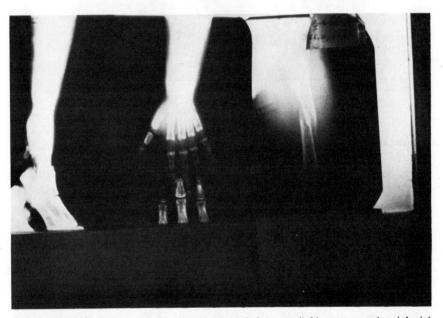

Figure 6. Rickets; X-ray changes showing healed fracture (left), metacarpal epiphysial dysplasia (center), active fracture (right).

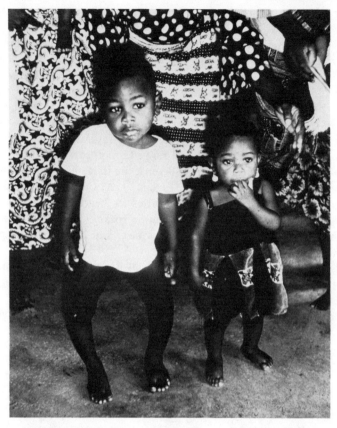

Figure 7. Rickets; bowing of lower extremities.

D-resistant rickets because it could not be satisfactorily treated even with massive doses of vitamin D—has remained a problem. In the last few years, our understanding of the metabolism of this vitamin has improved and, for the first time, specific therapy for certain forms of vitamin D-resistant rickets is possible. Recent investigations into the biochemical mechanisms for the action of vitamin D demonstrate, perhaps better than in any other area of nutrition, how fundamental research can have a direct and immediate influence on clinical practice.

Metabolism of Vitamin D

In the strict sense, cholecalciferol (vitamin D_3) is not a vitamin, since it can be synthesized in the presence of ultraviolet light from 7-dehydro-

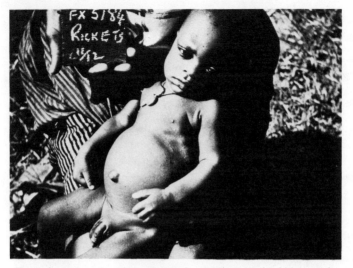

Figure 8. Rickets; knobbing of costochondral junction (rachitic rosary).

cholesterol, a normal component of skin. Therefore, an individual who is exposed to adequate amounts of sunlight does not require the vitamin. Vitamin D_3, whether synthesized in skin or supplied directly from the diet, must undergo a series of metabolic transformations before it reaches its active form (Figure 9). When absorbed through the gastrointestinal tract the vitamin is bound directly to chylomicrons and released into the general circulation.

In either case, vitamin D_3 is transformed in the liver to 25-hydroxy-cholecalciferol (25-HCC). In this form it is transported by an α-globulin to the kidney, where it is further hydroxylated to 1,25 dihydroxy-cholecalciferol (1,25-DCC), which is the active molecule. The 1,25-DCC acts on specific target tissues peripheral to its site of synthesis, and hence is a hormone. Vitamin D is a unique vitamin because it can be synthesized by the body in sunlight and because it is a hormone in its active form. In a sense, the vitamin's availability in food is a backup system for use when sunlight is not available.

Regulation and Mechanism of Action

The major actions of vitamin D are to promote intestinal absorption of calcium and phosphate and to mediate the mobilization of calcium from bone. In this manner, the vitamin helps to maintain blood calcium and phosphorus levels. Although there is some minimal physiologic activity in

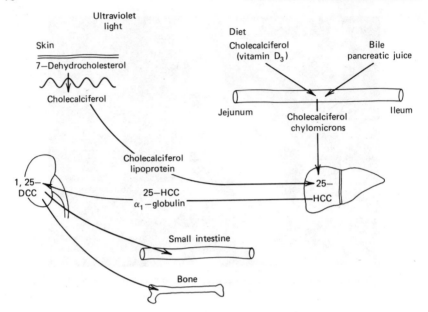

Figure 9. Pathway of vitamin D metabolism.

vitamin D_3 itself, and somewhat more in 25-HCC, which is made in the liver, by far the greatest activity is present in the 1,25-DCC derived from the kidney. This is the physiologically active hormone and the primary source of vitamin D activity in normal individuals.

The major regulation of vitamin D activity occurs in the kidney. There, the activity of 1 α-hydroxylase, the enzyme necessary for the final hydroxylation and conversion to the active form, is regulated by the individual's vitamin D and calcium status. Thus, animals made hypocalcemic by either a vitamin D-deficient or a calcium-deficient diet have increased renal 1 α-hydroxylase activity, which presumably produces more 1,25-DCC to correct the hypocalcemia by mobilizing calcium from the gut and the skeleton.

There is some evidence that hypophosphatemia as well as hypocalcemia may indirectly signal increased enzyme activity by changes in the levels of secreted or circulating parathyroid hormone. Available evidence suggests that parathyroid hormone, phosphate, vitamin D or one of its metabolites, and possibly calcium all play a role in regulating the synthesis of 1,25-DCC.

The mode of action of 1,25-DCC is currently under investigation. As previously suggested, 1,25-DCC mediates normal calcium metabolism and bone development and apparently can carry out all of the functions previously ascribed to vitamin D. Exactly how this is accomplished is not entirely understood. However, available data demonstrate that the stimulation of intestinal calcium transport by 1,25-DCC is due in part to an increased rate of calcium uptake by intestinal cells and in part to the formation of a specific calcium-binding protein (CaBP). Present data suggest that the hormone acts directly on the nucleus of the intestinal cell, unlocking a chain of events which ultimately leads to the synthesis of CaBP; CaBP, in turn, regulates the absorption of calcium from the gastrointestinal tract.

Assays have been, and still are being, developed for identifying the active vitamin D metabolites. These are now being used to identify patients with defects in vitamin D metabolism and to identify the cause of unexplained calcium abnormalities.

Two methods have been established for assaying the circulating amount of 25-HCC, the first conversion product that is synthesized in the liver. Both methods suggest normal levels of 20 to 30 ng/ml (5×10^{-8} M) in humans. Vitamin D_3 itself circulates at approximately the same levels. One important clinical finding that has resulted from the availability of this assay has been that epileptic patients on long-term therapy with phenytoin sodium (Dilantin[R]), phenobarbital, or both have lower than normal circulating concentrations of 25-HCC. This finding explains the high incidence of osteomalacia in such patients. The low blood levels of 25-HCC can be corrected by daily supplements of this vitamin D metabolite or by ingesting at least 4000 IU/week of vitamin D.

Recently, an assay has become available for measuring circulating levels of 1,25-DCC, the active hormone. The plasma level in normal man is 3 to 6 ng/100 ml, or about 1×10^{-10} M. This is one five-hundredth of the circulating concentration of either of the precursor sterols (vitamin D_3 or 25-HCC), and is in the same range as aldosterone, another steroid hormone.

The availability of this assay has enabled certain investigators to start probing the possibility that certain metabolic bone diseases are associated with abnormal circulating levels of 1,25-DCC. Because the hormone is synthesized in the kidney, initial studies have been undertaken in patients with renal disease. Available data indicate that patients with untreated renal failure have significantly reduced levels of 1,25-DCC. Moreover, the most striking reductions are found in patients with end-stage renal disease who have been on renal dialysis for as long as 4 years. In one anephrotic patient, levels of 1,25-DCC rose to normal within 3 weeks of successful renal transplant. These data strongly support the concept that, in humans,

1,25-DCC is synthesized exclusively in the kidney and that synthesis is interfered with in chronic renal disease, leading to the renal osteodystrophy and calcium imbalance seen in these patients.

In other studies, early indications suggest that levels of 1,25-DCC are slightly depressed in patients whose parathyroid gland has been removed or who have idiopathic hypoparathyroidism. Conversely, these levels are increased in patients with primary hyperparathyroidism. Hence, parathyroid hormone may be an important factor influencing the synthesis and secretion of 1,25-DCC in man.

Therapeutic Advances

These observations have lead to rapid progress in therapy for a number of heretofore poorly controlled diseases. Patients with chronic renal disease have been successfully treated with 1,25-DCC, and there is evidence that long-term administration of this hormone in such patients can reverse both the osteitis fibrosa cystica and the osteomalacia associated with renal disease. Another therapeutic advance has been the discovery that patients with vitamin D-resistant rickets will respond to doses of 1,25-DCC as low as 1 μg. This suggests that the genetic abnormality in this disease occurs in the synthesis or secretion of 1,25-DCC.

By contrast, hypophosphatemic vitamin D-resistant rickets, another inherited disorder resulting in osteomalacia which is refractory to normal doses of vitamin D, apparently cannot be corrected by treatment with 1,25-DCC. It has therefore been postulated that this disease is the result of faulty renal phosphate transport rather than defective production of the hormone. Finally, patients with hypoparathyroidism previously resistant to 400,000 IU (10 mg)/day of vitamin D have responded to oral doses of 1,25-DCC as low as 1 μg/day. Hence this hormone represents a much more powerful agent for correcting the low serum calcium levels and preventing tetany in these patients.

As we further unravel the mysteries of vitamin D metabolism we can expect rapid progress in our understanding of certain metabolic bone diseases and in our ability to treat certain patients previously doomed to a life of chronic debilitating diseases which progressed, in spite of therapy, to early death.

These studies in vitamin D metabolism highlight the dramatic differences in medical priorities within the world. In developing countries, rickets is due to lack of exposure to sunlight and to faulty diet. The treatment is obvious, yet even extensive public health measures have not eliminated the disease. In developed countries, where primary rickets is no longer a problem, genetic forms of this disease, endocrine abnormalities resulting in rickets, and the rickets or osteomalacia of renal disease, all extremely rare diseases by comparison, are now being understood and in the near future should be brought under control.

VITAMIN E DEFICIENCY

Vitamin E (α-tocopherol) is currently gaining notoriety as a potential panacea. It is being marketed with exaggerated claims, including the suggestion that it increases libido and sexual potency both in males and in females. It is interesting that with all of these claims, human vitamin E deficiency has been extremely hard to produce in adult volunteers and deficiency symptoms rarely occur in children or adults except in severe cases of malabsorption, such as cystic fibrosis. However, in premature infants a specific syndrome due to vitamin E deficiency has been described. Several authors have reported symptoms of irritability and edema accompanied by anemia in premature infants who were consuming formulas containing inadequate amounts of vitamin E. The anemia that accompanies vitamin E deficiency in premature infants is hemolytic in nature, resulting in a shortened life span of the red cell. It does not respond to iron and, in fact, iron therapy may aggravate the anemia. By contrast, this anemia can be cured by the administration of vitamin E. Since premature infants have extremely limited vitamin E stores, in part because of their limited amount of adipose tissue, where vitamin E is stored, the deficiency develops rapidly. By contrast, in the adult, the one depletion study that was carried out over a long time demonstrated that after 3 years, although plasma tocopherol fell to very low levels, no symptoms developed. A slight decrease in red cell life span was found, but there was no anemia.

Even in patients with severe malabsorption syndromes who have low blood levels of the vitamin, no symptoms that can be corrected with vitamin E alone have been reported. Recently, however, there is a preliminary report that the abnormal sweat electrolytes in children with cystic fibrosis can be brought toward normal by prolonged treatment with vitamin E.

Tocopherols, which form the class of compounds that have vitamin E activity, are found associated with the lipid fractions of many plants and animals and hence are widely available in the diet. Although α-tocopherol is the most active compound, other members of this class, such as γ-tocopherol, can contribute significant amounts of vitamin E activity from the diet. As United States diets move in the direction of more vegetable fats and oils and less animal fat, the importance of the γ derivative becomes greater.

The metabolism of vitamin E is not fully worked out. Figure 10 is a

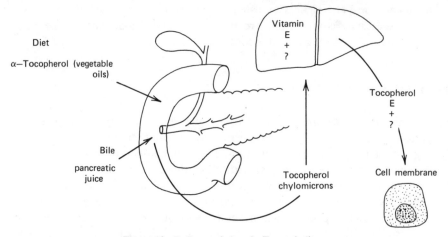

Figure 10. Pathway of vitamin E metabolism.

schematic representation of events as they are currently understood. The tocopherols from animal or vegetable sources are absorbed in the small intestine after exposure to bile and pancreatic juices. In man only about 20 to 30% of α-tocopherol is absorbed at low doses and probably less at higher doses. Vitamin E is transported, bound to chylomicrons, to the liver, where it is either stored or released into the general circulation. The form in which it is stored and the way it is transported in the plasma are not known. What is known from experimental work in animals and a few studies in humans, is that vitamin E is stored in most tissues, with the largest amount stored in the adipose tissue. In depletion studies, when the vitamin is removed from the diet, almost one-half of the α-tocopherol in liver and heart was lost in 2 weeks, with the remainder disappearing over a long period of time. Other tissues, with the exception of the adipose depot, also seem to have two pools of stored vitamin E, the first released relatively rapidly, the second depleted much more slowly and postulated to represent α-tocopherol in cellular membranes.

The method of transport of vitamin E in the plasma is not fully understood and to date no specific protein carrier has been found analogous to the carrier proteins for some of the other fat-soluble vitamins. What is known is that tocopherols in plasma are associated with the lipoproteins and are distributed in proportion to the fat content of each fraction. Plasma tocopherol levels correlate with plasma cholesterol or total lipid levels. Thus, plasma tocopherol levels in themselves probably have little meaning if not accompanied by values for plasma lipids. A ratio of 0.8 mg of total tocopherols per gram of total lipids has been suggested as a value demonstrating adequate nutritional status for vitamin E. If this ratio is used instead of the previously accepted absolute value of 0.5 mg/100 ml of blood, many patients who were considered deficient actually would not be. It is also possible that certain individuals with high serum lipids may have adequate amounts with a ratio of less than 0.8 mg of tocopherols per gram of lipid.

The search for the mode of action of vitamin E at the tissue and cellular levels is the main area of current research with this vitamin. Many studies have attempted to demonstrate a direct effect of this vitamin on the function of certain enzymes. Recently attention has focused on two enzymes involved in heme synthesis. Vitamin E depletion resulted in a reduced activity of δ-aminolevulinic acid (ALA) synthetase in bone marrow and a reduced activity of ALA dehydratase in liver. However, other studies have failed to demonstrate any effect of vitamin E deficiency on the actual rate of heme synthesis. Hence, at present, there is no conclusive evidence for a regulatory role of vitamin E in hemoglobin or cytochrome synthesis.

It has been demonstrated that in vitamin E-deficient rats, the microsomal enzyme drug-hydroxylating complex is reduced and can be restored within 12 hours of the administration of vitamin E by mouth. This complex, however, is hormone sensitive and hence the mechanism by which vitamin E produces its effect is unknown. At present, then, it has not been demonstrated that any enzyme reaction is specifically affected by vitamin E.

Another role that has been postulated for vitamin E is as an antioxidant. In this manner, it is believed to stabilize lipid membranes in a variety of tissues. In addition, it may protect against certain environmental pollutants. Supplementary α-tocopherol has been shown to offer protection from an experimental high oxygen atmosphere and, more recently, protection from ozone and nitrous oxide have been demonstrated. All of these gases can cause lipid peroxidation damage in rat tissues, but the relevance of these results to man is not clear. In man, there are other protective mechanisms against lipid peroxidation in the lung; for example, the activity of glucose-6-phosphate dehydrogenase, of glutathione peroxidase, and of superoxide dismutase. Thus, the relative importance and effectiveness of α-tocopherol as a tissue antioxidant in man remains unclear.

From the foregoing discussion it should be quite clear that except in the premature infant there is no specific human deficiency disease caused by a lack of vitamin E. In addition, although vitamin E has been shown to affect certain metabolic processes, there is as yet no specific role for vitamin E in human metabolism. For these reasons it is impossible to set human requirements in a manner similar to the way requirements are set for other vitamins, that is, the amount necessary to prevent deficiency symptoms plus a safety factor. The recommended dietary allowance for vitamin E has therefore been estimated by determining the range of vitamin E present in a variety of diets that are adequate for all other nutrients. With this method 10 to 20 IU of total vitamin E activity were recommended for healthy young adults. While it was pointed out that this is probably not a realistic amount for growing children and during other critical periods of life, such as pregnancy and adolescence, it is reasonable for anyone consuming 1800 to 3000 cal/day. These values must be considered approximations and averages which may or may not be adequate depending on other components of the diet, primarily polyunsaturated fatty acid (PUFA) content. However, under most circumstances, as the PUFA in diets increases, so does the vitamin E content.

Since the recommended allowance is based on the amount of vitamin E in balanced diets, it is extremely important that vitamin E levels in food be accurately determined. Newer analytical methods have demonstrated that the average American or Canadian diet contains 6.4 to 9.0 mg (9.5 to 13.4 IU) of α-tocopherol daily. In addition, United States diets now contain considerably more γ-tocopherol than α-tocopherol, since the former is present in six times the amount of the latter in soybean oil, which is the vegetable oil most consumed in the United States. Although the γ form is less active than the α form, it currently makes up to 20 to 30% of the total vitamin E activity in the American diet. In addition, other vitomers, such as β-tocopherol and α-tocotreinol, which are found in whole cereal grains, also contribute to the available vitamin E. For this reason, total vitamin E requirements are expressed in α-tocopherol equivalents, which are derived by multiplying the amount of α-tocopherol by 1.2 (to allow for the other forms of the vitamin that are less active but present in significant amounts).

Vitamin E still remains in some ways a "vitamin in search of a disease." Although deficiency states can be demonstrated clearly under certain conditions, and frank disease may occur in depleted premature infants, primary deficiency of this vitamin is very rare. Whether this is due to its widespread distribution in foods or to our inability to recognize subclinical disease is unknown. From the foregoing evidence it is difficult to see how this vitamin has gotten its reputation as a cure-all. Objective evidence of beneficial effects of large doses of vitamin E in the human is lacking. In animals certain toxic effects of large doses have been observed. Toxicity of vitamins will be dealt with in Chapter 15, but it should be noted that in man, relatively high doses of vitamin E (300 IU daily) appear safe in the short run. However, we have no idea what the long-term consequences of such large doses of this vitamin, stored in considerable amounts by the body, might be.

VITAMIN K DEFICIENCY

Our major sources of vitamin K are green leafy vegetables (e.g., broccoli, lettuce, cabbage, and spinach) and red meat, particularly beef liver. All forms of vitamin K belong to the naphthoquinone family of compounds.

Vitamin K is absorbed from the small intestine after exposure to bile and pancreatic juices. Bound to chylomicrons, it is then transported to the liver, which either stores it or releases it into the bloodstream, where it circulates attached to β-lipoproteins (Figure 11).

Vitamin K's one known physiologic role is as a cofactor in synthesizing the various proteins needed for blood clotting, the most important being prothrombin.

Since many bacteria, including E. coli, synthesize vitamin K, primary deficiency almost never occurs in adults. It does occur in newborn infants, however, because of their sterile gastrointestinal tracts and the fact that both breast milk and cow's milk contain little vitamin K. Since affected infants may experience uncontrolled bleeding, many hospitals now give prophylactic vitamin K to all newborns within hours of delivery. Vitamin K is also the treatment of choice for infants already affected.

Secondary vitamin K deficiency occurs primarily in patients with biliary obstruction or severe malabsorptive disease, or in those receiving total parenteral nutrition without added vitamin K.

In addition to reversing deficiency states, vitamin K is used to counter the effects of anticoagulants like dicoumarol. It is given if and when anticoagulant therapy causes bleeding.

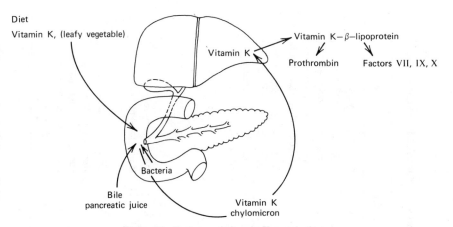

Figure 11. Pathway of vitamin K metabolism.

Table 3. Fat-soluble vitamins

Vitamin	Source	Transport	Action	Deficiency	Excess
A	Diet—meat, butter, egg yolk, fatty fish (retinol), green and yellow vegetables (carotene); recommended intake 5000 IU/day adult	RBP Prealbumin	Activates rhodopsin, maintains epithelial integrity	Night blindness Squamous metaplasia Xerophthalmia Keratosis	Drowsiness, intracranial pressure, vomiting, peeling of skin
D	Diet—fish oils, egg yolks, margarine; skin, and ultraviolet light; recommended intake 400 IU/day	α-Globulin	Converted into a steroid hormone by two step hydroxylation Hormone: stimulates calcium absorption and bone deposition	Rickets Osteomalacia	Nausea, vomiting, thirst, polyuria, stupor, coma, metastatic calcification
K	Diet—leafy vegetables Bacterial synthesis	β-Lipoprotein	Activates prothrombin Factor VII, IX, X	Bleeding	
E	Diet—vegetables, oils, margarine, shortening, eggs, butter, wholemeal cereals, broccoli; recommended intake 15 IU/day		Maintainance of cell membranes	Red cell hemolysis	

Table 3 summarizes the dietary sources, transport, action, and major signs of deficiency and excess of the four fat-soluble vitamins.

RECOMMENDED READING

Aballi, A. J., The Action of Vitamin K in the Neonatal Period, *Southern Med. J.,* **58,** (1), 48 (1965).

Avioli, L. V., and J. C. Haddad, Vitamin D: Current Concepts, *Metabolism,* **22,** 507 (1973).

Bieri, J. G., Fat-Soluble Vitamins in the Eighth Revision of the Recommended Dietary Allowances, *J. Am. Diet. Assoc.,* **64,** 171 (1974).

Bieri, J. G., Vitamin E, *Nutr. Rev.,* **33,** 161 (1975).

Davis, K., Vitamin E, Adequacy of Infants' Diets, *Am. J. Clin. Nutr.,* **25,** 933 (1975).

De Luca, H. F., Vitamin D, A New Look at an Old Vitamin, *Nutr. Rev.,* **29,** 179 (1971).

De Luca, H. F., Vitamin D-Resistant Rickets, A Prototype of Nutritional Management of a Genetic Disorder, in M. Winick, Ed., *Nutritional Management of Genetic Disorders,* Wiley, New York, 1979, pp. 3–32.

De Luca, H. F., and J. W. Sutlie, Eds., *The Fat-Soluble Vitamins,* University of Wisconsin Press, Madison, 1970.

Draper, H. H., and A. S. Callany, Metabolism and Function of Vitamin E, *Fed. Proc.,* **28,** 1690 (1969).

Fomon, S. J., M. K. Younoszai, and L. N. Thomas, Influence of Vitamin D on Linear Growth of Normal Full-Term Infants, *J. Nutr.,* **88,** 345 (1966).

Goldman, H. I., and P. Amades, Vitamin K Deficiency after the Newborn Period, *Pediatrics,* **44,** 745 (1969).

Goodman, D. S., Biosynthesis of Vitamin A from β-Carotene, *Am. J. Clin. Nutr.,* **22,** 963 (1969).

Kodicek, E., The Story of Vitamin D From Vitamin to Hormone, *Lancet,* **1,** 325 (1974).

Leonard, P. J., and M. S. Losowsky, Effect of Alphatocopherol Administration on Red Cell Survival in Vitamin E-Deficient Human Subjects, *Am. J. Clin. Nutr.,* **24,** 388 (1971).

Nammacher, M. A., M. Willemin, J. 'Hartmann, and L. Gaslon, Vitamin K Deficiency in Infants Beyond the Neonatal Period, *J. Pediat.,* **76,** 549 (1970).

Olson, R. E., Vitamin E and its Relation to Heart Disease, *Circulation,* **48,** 179 (1973).

Oomen, H. A. P. C., Vitamin A Deficiency, Xerophthalmia; and Blindness, in *Present Knowledge in Nutrition,* The Nutrition Foundation, Washington, D. C., 1976.

Rodriguez, M. E., and M. L. Irwin, A Conceptus of Research on Vitamin A Requirements in Man, *J. Nutr.,* **102,** 909 (1972).

Roels, O. A., Vitamin A Physiology, *JAMA,* **214,** 1097, (1970).

Sutlie, J. W., Vitamin K and Prothrombin Synthesis, *Nutr. Rev.,* **31,** 105 (1973).

Vitamin A, Xerophthalmia and Blindness, A.I.D. Report, U.S. State Dept. (1973).

Witting, L. A., Recommended Dietary Allowance for Vitamin E, *Am. J. Clin. Nutr.,* **25,** 257 (1972).

Wolf, G., International Symposium on Metabolic Function of Vitamin A, *Am. J. Clin. Nutr.,* **22,** 903 (1969).

9

DEFICIENCIES OF
WATER-SOLUBLE
VITAMINS

The water-soluble vitamins include ascorbic acid (vitamin C) and a group of B complex vitamins, thiamin (B_1), niacin, riboflavin, pyridoxine (B_6), pantothenic acid, biotin, folic acid, and cyanocobalamin (B_{12}). None of these vitamins is stored in any appreciable quantities in the body and hence they are required in regular amounts throughout life. Because excess amounts of the water-soluble vitamins are rapidly excreted in the urine, they are much less toxic than the fat-soluble vitamins. The amount of time necessary to produce deficiency will vary from one vitamin to another. In the human infant B_6 deficiency can develop very rapidly, in a matter of days. By contrast, B_{12} deficiency, except in the very young, often takes years to develop.

The conquest of the various water-soluble vitamin deficiencies, which took place in the early part of the 20th century, is one of the most exciting chapters in all medical history. It demonstrated, perhaps more clearly than had ever been demonstrated before, how a biochemical discovery could lead to the cure of a disease and conversely how an empirically successful treatment could lead to a biochemical discovery. This chapter will attempt to outline the most important aspects of the action of the water-soluble vitamins, the clinical manifestations of deficiency, and the use of these vitamins in therapy. In addition, a discussion of inborn errors of vitamin metabolism is included. The use and misuse of vitamins and minerals in our society will be discussed at the end of Chapter 10.

ASCORBIC ACID (VITAMIN C)

The major sources of vitamin C are fruits, especially citrus fruits, and vege-tables, including potatoes. The classic disease caused by vitamin C deficiency is scurvy, which is manifested by changes in the gums and abnormal bleeding into skin, subcutaneous tissue, and even below the periosteum of bone. The gums are swollen, particularly in the regions of the papillae between the teeth, sometimes producing the appearance of "scurvy buds." These may be so extensive that they project beyond the biting surface of the teeth and almost completely conceal them. The swollen gums are livid in color and bleed at the slightest touch. There is always some infection and often a strikingly offensive odor. In patients without teeth, however, the gums appear normal.

Cutaneous bleeding often begins on the lower thighs as perifollicular hemorrhages, which may then spread to the buttocks, abdomen, legs, and arms. Petechial hemorrhages may also appear as a result of rupture of capillary vessels. Thereafter, large spontaneous bruises (ecchymoses) may arise almost anywhere in the body. In addition, ocular hemorrhages, drying of salivary and lachrymal glands, parotid swelling, femoral neuropathy, edema of the lower extremities, and psychological disturbances have been described. Patients with scurvy may also develop anemia, may display radiologic changes of osteoporosis, and may die suddenly, presumably from heart failure.

Although scurvy was one of the earliest described of the vitamin diseases and although the essential nutrient ascorbic acid was identified early in this century, the exact metabolic role of vitamin C is still unclear. This is probably the main reason for the controversy that rages around the use of the vitamin. Ascorbic acid is important in collagen formation and is in some way involved in the growth of fibroblasts, osteoblasts, and odonto-blasts, as well as in the hydroxylation of proline and lysine. It may play a role in wound healing and in the formation of some of the neurotrans-mitters. Ascorbic acid is a potent reducing agent, thus enhancing iron absorption and inhibiting copper absorption.

The normal requirement for vitamin C has become a very controversial subject. Certainly amounts in the range suggested as the RDA (40 mg/day) are adequate not only to cure scurvy and prevent any signs from recurring, but also for maintaining good health at least from the standpoint of obvious pathology or pathophysiology. Recent data suggest that heavy smokers have lower blood levels of circulating vitamin C and may therefore have somewhat higher requirements. The disagreement relates to whether much larger quantities are necessary to prevent more subtle changes in body function. This entire issue of the use of "megadoses" of vitamins in the quest for "optimal" health is discussed in Chapter 15.

VITAMIN B$_1$ (THIAMIN)

Thiamin or vitamin B$_1$ is found in large amounts in bran, yeast, and whole grain cereals, as well as in smaller amounts in fresh fruits and vegetables and most meats and fish. Eighty percent of the thiamin in the body is in the form of thiamin pyrophosphate (TPP), 10% is in the form of thiamin triphosphate (TTP), and the remainder is in the form of thiamin monophosphate (TMP), or free thiamin. Thiamin pyrophosphate functions as a coenzyme in the oxidative decarboxylation of alpha-keto acids and also as a transketolase in the pentose phosphate shunt. Thus it has a central role in both carbohydrate and amino acid metabolism. In addition, it has an independent role in neurophysiology which has not been clearly defined.

Deficiency of vitamin B$_1$ can be primary and still is widespread in poor rural Asian populations that subsist mainly on polished rice. In more developed countries, including the United States, secondary deficiency may be encountered. In alcoholics, especially those in a state of chronic malnutrition, intestinal absorption of thiamin may be impaired and symptoms of frank deficiency may develop.

Primary deficiency results in beriberi, which may occur in one of three forms: (1) wet beriberi, characterized by edema often associated with high output cardiac failure, (2) dry beriberi, a polyneuropathy, and (3) the infantile form. Infantile beriberi is still a leading cause of death between the ages of 2 and 5 months in rice-eating rural areas. It may be acute, with edema, cyanosis, cardiac failure, and death, or it may be chronic, with mainly gastrointestinal symptoms. In very severe cases the infant may become partially or completely aphonic.

Secondary thiamin deficiency, seen mainly in alcoholics, is often accompanied by other nutritional deficiencies and therefore may not present as pure beriberi. Nevertheless both the wet and dry forms are encountered. In the wet form the patient may rapidly develop heart failure, with edema, pulmonary congestion, dyspnea, cardiomegaly, and signs of high cardiac output, such as warm skin and bounding pulse. Fifty to one hundred mg of thiamin, administered intramuscularly, will rapidly correct the condition. Thus in any patient with unexplained high output cardiac failure, especially one who has a history of alcoholism, a therapeutic trial of thiamin is indicated and may be life saving. Figure 1 shows the cardiomegaly associated with beriberi and the dramatic response to therapy.

Alcoholic polyneuropathy is most often due to thiamin deficiency, al-

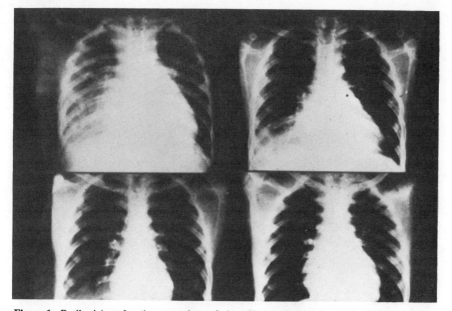

Figure 1. Beriberi (wet form); comparison of chest X-rays showing heart size before thiamin treatment (upper left) and response to therapy measured at 10 day intervals (clockwise).

though deficiencies in other vitamins can cause identical symptoms. The lesions are symmetrical and the nerves of the lower limbs are affected more severely than the nerves of the upper limbs. Both motor and sensory fibers are involved. Signs of motor nerve involvement include wrist and foot drop (Figure 2) muscle wasting, and impaired knee and ankle jerks. The signs of sensory nerve involvement may include paresthesias, severe nerve pains, loss of sensation, numbness, and loss of position sense.

Another syndrome resulting from thiamin deficiency, and again seen primarily but not exclusively in alcoholics, is the Wernicke-Korsakoff syndrome. This may begin with nystagmus, eye muscle weakness, ataxia, disorientation, and apathy, and may progress to frank psychosis characterized by short-term memory defects, confabulation, and learning defects. In this syndrome, early diagnosis is important since to be effective thiamin must be given in the same large doses as for wet beriberi, early in the course of the disease.

NIACIN (NICOTINIC ACID)

The classic niacin deficiency disease is pellagra. It is endemic among poor peasants who subsist chiefly on maize. The typical clinical features

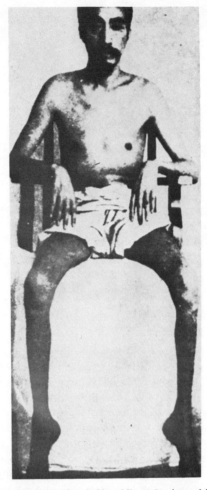

Figure 2. Beriberi (dry form). Note bilateral wrist and foot drop.

are loss of weight, increasing debility, an erythematous dermatitis characteristically affecting parts of the skin exposed to sunlight, gastrointestinal
disturbance, especially diarrhea, glossitis and mental changes. Although
formerly quite prevalent in the south, at present pellagra is rarely seen
in the United States.

Nicotinamide is a component of certain respiratory coenzymes and is
therefore concerned with tissue oxidation. The human body is not entirely
dependent on dietary sources of nicotinic acid, since the vitamin may be
synthesized from the essential amino acid tryptophan. Sixty mg of dietary

tryptophan are necessary to replace 1 mg of niacin. Hence it is better to talk about the niacin equivalent in food (niacin plus one sixtieth of the tryptophan content). Thus, although milk and eggs are poor sources of niacin, they have a high niacin equivalent. Niacin is widely distributed in plant and animal foods, but in relatively small amounts. Meats (especially organs), fish, whole grain cereals, and pulses are good sources of niacin. As a result of this widespread distribution even a moderately good diet should easily supply the 6.6 mg/1000 kcal of niacin equivalents that constitute the recommended daily allowance.

RIBOFLAVIN

Riboflavin is a yellow-green fluorescent compound which is a major component of important coenzymes concerned with tissue oxidation. Severe deficiency can result in angular stomatitis, cheilosis, nasolabial seborrhea (seen in Figure 3), and invasion of the cornea by capillaries accompanied by lachrymation and photophobia.

In view of the importance of riboflavin in cell respiration it is surprising that the clinical symptoms of deficiency are minor and do not themselves threaten life. Even though riboflavin has a wide distribution in foodstuffs, many people live for long periods on very low intake and consequently

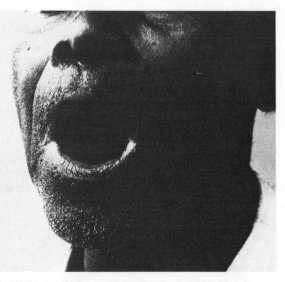

Figure 3. Riboflavin deficiency. Cheilosis and nasolabial seborrhea.

minor signs of deficiency are common in many parts of the world. This is probably true among poorer populations in the United States, who have been shown in surveys to tend to have low blood levels. Why these conditions do not progress and lead to serious illness remains a mystery.

The best sources of riboflavin are liver, milk, eggs, and green vegetables. It differs from other B complex vitamins in that it is present in good amounts in dairy products but in only small amounts in cereal grains. It is also present in beer.

PYRIDOXINE (VITAMIN B$_6$)

Vitamin B$_6$ and its metabolites are essential for a number of important metabolic reactions including transamination, porphyrin and heme synthesis, and the conversion of tryptophan to niacin.

Although primary dietary deficiency is probably rare, secondary deficiencies due to increased requirements either genetically induced or environmentally imposed are commonly encountered. Convulsions or chronic anemia can occur in infants with different types of genetic diseases which respond to large doses of vitamin B$_6$.

The antituberculosis drug Isoniazid is a vitamn B$_6$ antagonist and can produce in patients being treated with it a peripheral neuropathy which can be prevented by giving 10 mg/day of pyridoxine. Another clinically useful drug, penicillamine, used in the treatment of Wilson's disease, cystinuria, and rheumatoid arthritis, also acts as a pyridoxine antagonist. Patients treated with penicillamine show abnormal tryptophan metabolism, and convulsions have been reported in a number of such patients. These symptoms can be completely prevented by vitamin B$_6$ supplementation.

Some women taking oral contraceptives become pyridoxine deficient judged by biochemical criteria. This deficiency may be due to an increased pyridoxine requirement. Such women may become depressed, and in some cases the depression disappears when pyridoxine (20 mg twice daily) is given.

In the above four conditions in which pyridoxine deficiency develops and is reversed by large doses of the vitamin, the presenting clinical features are, respectively, anemia, failure to thrive, peripheral neuropathy, and depression. These are common conditions and in most cases are certainly not due to pyridoxine deficiency. However, when one of these features is present, there is no obvious cause, and all other remedies have failed, a therapeutic trial of pyridoxine may be considered. No adverse reaction has been reported to such administration.

Vitamin B_6 is widely distributed in animal and plant tissues and is found in large amounts in meats, vegetables, and bran. Most human diets provide 1 to 2 mg/day, which is certainly sufficient for most people.

PANTOTHENIC ACID

Pantothenic acid is a constituent of coenzyme A and is present in all living matter. Its distribution in natural foodstuffs is so widespread that deficiency of the vitamin is unlikely to occur in man except perhaps when unenriched highly processed foods are consumed almost exclusively.

BIOTIN

Except for a few reported cases in individuals with very bizarre eating habits, biotin deficiency does not occur in man. Yeasts and many bacteria either make or retain biotin. It seems probable that man can obtain all he needs from the numerous microorganisms that are present in foods, or in his own large intestines. In addition, certain foods, for example, egg, liver, kidney, pulses, nuts, chocolate, and some vegetables, are rich in biotin. The human body utilizes a few micrograms of biotin daily.

FOLIC ACID

Folate coenzymes participate in a number of essential metabolic reactions, including purine and thymidylate biosynthesis, and hence in the synthesis of DNA, and they are important in the metabolism of certain amino acids. In this last respect, the remethylation of homocysteine to methionine is particularly important, since methionine serves as the methyl donor for a large number of methylation reactions. Only bacteria and plants can synthesize folic acid and hence in all animals it must be supplied in the diet. The best source of this vitamin is liver. However, significant amounts are present in lentils, beans, and orange and grapefruit juice, as well as in most vegetables and various types of seafood, including oysters and white fish. In addition, whole grain bread, products using enriched flour, and various meats and eggs are moderately good sources of folic acid.

Most naturally occurring folate is in a nonactive form and must be cleaved in the intestinal cells during the process of absorption. Once this is accomplished, active folate enters the bloodstream, circulates to the liver, and continues from there to the peripheral tissues.

The main metabolic consequence of folic acid deficiency is a derangement of DNA synthesis and consequently a slowing down or arrest in cell division. This effect is easily understood in view of the aforementioned essential role of folate in the biosynthesis of thymidylate and of purines. The result is a set of characteristic changes in nuclear morphology. Tissues having the highest rate of cell multiplication are affected first. These predominantly nuclear alterations are referred to as "megaloblastic," a term usually applied to the nucleated cells in the red cell series in bone marrow. However, morphological changes can also be seen in the nuclei of leukocytes as well as in the epithelial cells of the stomach, small intestine, vagina, and uterine cervix.

Thus folic acid deficiency, no matter what the cause, results in anemia with all of its attendant signs and symptoms: pallor, lethargy, weakness, and a lowered hemoglobin concentration. The anemia is macrocytic and hypochromic, and the bone marrow shows a characterisitc megaloblatosis (Figure 4).

Primary folic acid deficiency due to an inadequate intake is probably the most common vitamin deficiency in man, especially in poorer populations. An intake of 50 mg of pteroylglutamic acid is the minimum amount of folate necessary to correct a state of pure deficiency, and 400 mg/day has been set as the RDA for a healthy adult. Any physiologic or pathologic

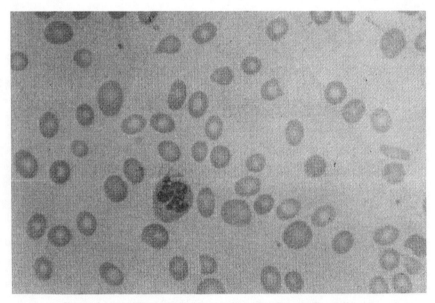

Figure 4. Megaloblastic anemia of folic acid or vitamin B$_{12}$ deficiency.

condition leading to increased rates of cell mulitplication will result in higher folic acid requirements. Thus pregnancy, lactation, early infancy, and adolescence are physiological states particularly vulnerable to the development of deficiency. Anemias of various origins, especially hemolytic anemias, malignancy, parasitic infestations, infection, and even aseptic abscesses also result in higher folate needs. Malabsorption of dietary folate occurs in gluten-induced enteropathy and in tropical sprue, but the underlying mechanisms are unknown.

A number of substances interfere with the normal absorption of folate, the most important of which is ethanol. Alcohol seems to affect not only folate absorption but also its metabolism. Hence, folic acid deficiency is a common complication in chronic alcoholism. Certain anticonvulsive drugs, in particular diphenylhydantoin, interfere with the absorption of free folic acid as well as with certain aspects of its metabolism. Patients being treated with such drugs may become deficient in folate and may require supplementation.

Inadequate utilization of folates is most often due to drugs that interfere with some aspects of folate metabolism. Methotrexate and other 4-amino-4-deoxyfolate analogs owe their antitumor effect to a potent inhibition in one of the early steps in the conversion of folic acid to its active coenzyme. This leads to eventual cell death. The margin between therapeutic and toxic doses is a narrow one, which is sometimes voluntarily overstepped. This has been advocated in therapeutic schemes designed to deliver massive doses of the drug to the tumor followed by "rescue" doses of N^5-formyl tetrahydrofolic acid that act as an antidote for the normal cells. It should be noted that these drugs are used not only in the treatment of malignancies but also in the treatment of psoriasis and as immunosuppressants, greatly increasing the number of people at risk from drug induced deficiency. In addition, other commonly used antifolates, such as the antimalarial drug pyrimethamine, the antibacterial drug trimethoprim, and the diuretic agent triamterene, may also interfere with folate metabolism.

There are several reports that oral contraceptive agents alter folate metabolism, primarily affecting the target organs themselves. Megaloblastic changes limited to the cervicovaginal epithelium may occur. Finally, the megaloblastic anemia of scurvy is clearly associated with a defect in the utilization of folates, the exact nature of which remains unknown.

VITAMIN B$_{12}$ (CYANOCOBALAMIN)

The only clearly delineated action of vitamin B$_{12}$ is to make active folate available for certain essential metabolic reactions. An enzyme containing vitamin B_{12} removes the methyl group from methyl folate, thereby regenerating tetrahydrofolate (THF), from which 5,10-methlylene THF is made and is then used in the synthesis of thymidylate. Since methyl folate is the predominant form of the vitamin in human serum and liver, and since methyl folate returns to the body's folate pool only via the vitamin B_{12}-dependent step, B_{12} deficiency results in folate's being "trapped" as methyl folate and thus becoming metabolically useless. Hence cyanocobalamin (B_{12}) is a vitamin that is essential for the proper utilization of another vitamin, folic acid. This interrelation between vitamin B_{12} and folic acid has been again demonstrated by the discovery that vitamin B_{12} is necessary for proper uptake of folate by cells. The "folate trap" hypothesis explains the fact that the hematologic changes in B_{12} deficiency are indistinguishable from those of folic acid deficiency. In both instances the defective synthesis of DNA results from a defect in the same final common pathway, namely, inadequate amounts of 5,10-methylene THF. Thus the cardinal finding in B_{12} deficiency is macrocytic hypochromic anemia with a megaloblastic marrow clinically and hematologically indistinguishable from the macrocytic hypochromic megaloblastic anemia of folic acid deficiency.

However, prolonged vitamin B_{12} deficiency produces changes in the central nervous system not seen in folate deficiency. This condition is characterized by patchy, diffuse, and progressive demyelination. The clinical picture is one of insidiously progressive neuropathy, often beginning in the peripheral nerves and progressing centrally to involve the posterior and lateral columns of the spinal cord and finally the brain itself. The neurological consequences of vitamin B_{12} deficiency are known by a variety of names: "subacute combined degeneration," or "combined system disease," or "posterior lateral sclerosis" when the spinal cord is involved, and "megaloblastic madness" when the brain is affected. Although certain defects in the fatty acids of myelin in patients with vitamin B_{12} deficiency have been described, the mechanism responsible for the demyelination is unknown.

Thus vitamin B_{12} seems to have an essential role independent of its role in folate metabolism. This is extremely important since treatment of the megaloblastic anemia of B_{12} deficiency with folic acid will entirely reverse the blood and bone marrow changes but will have no effect on the neurological disease, which will progress unabated. It is therefore extremely important, when confronted with a megaloblastic anemia, to make the proper etiologic diagnosis and institute *specific* therapy.

All vitamin B_{12} found in nature is made by microorganisms. Therefore, it is absent in plants except in the root nodules of certain legumes which are contaminated by microorganisms. Fruits, vegetables, grains, and grain products are all devoid of vitamin B_{12}. Fecal material contains B_{12}-synthesizing organisms; however, since the vitamin is not absorbed from the colon, strict vegetarians always develop vitamin B_{12} deficiency slowly over a period of many years. Delay in the development of vitamin B_{12} deficiency in strictly vegetarian children may relate in part to cleanliness; the less thoroughly they wash their hands after defecation, the more frequently they suck their fingers, the more they protect themselves against developing B_{12} deficiency. The usual dietary sources of vitamin B_{12} are meat and meat products, including shellfish, fish, poultry, and eggs, and to a lesser extent milk and milk products. Particularly rich sources of vitamin B_{12} include organ meats, such as lamb and beef liver, kidney, and heart, and bivalves, such as clams and oysters. Moderate amounts are present in nonfat dry milk, certain seafood, and egg yolks, and to a lesser extent in muscle meats and fermented cheese.

The recommended dietary intake of vitamin B_{12} is 3 mg/day for a healthy adult; during pregnancy or lactation the RDA increases to 4 mg/day. For normal B_{12} absorption the stomach must be functioning properly, since gastric acid helps free B_{12} from its tight protein bonds in food, and the gastric parietal cells secrete a glycoprotein called intrinsic factor (IF), which is essential for B_{12} absorption from the ileum. In addition, the pancreas must secrete adequate amounts of trypsin and bicarbonate, which facilitate B_{12} absorption, and there must be an intact ileum across whose cells B_{12} is absorbed into the circulation. Although primary vitamin B_{12} deficiency is not common except in very strict vegetarians, secondary deficiency is commonly encountered. Total gastric resection requires parenteral B_{12} injections. One hundred micrograms injected once a month will totally protect against deficiency. Less frequently pancreatic disease or severe ileal disease may necessitate similar therapy. Since B_{12} deficiency takes a long time to manifest itself (sometimes several years) physicians must remain alert for potential situations in which it might occur.

GENETIC DISEASES OF VITAMIN METABOLISM

Although vitamins are essential nutrients, they must be absorbed, transported in the plasma, enter target cells, compartmentalize within the cell, convert to an active coenzyme form, and finally attach to an apoenzyme to form the holoenzyme which catalyzes a particular reaction. Each of these six steps requires at least one particular type of protein in order to be carried out. In a genetic sense there are potentially six separate loci on which a mutation can derange normal vitamin metabolism. Depending on the particular locus, the manifestation of the altered metabolism will differ. Thus if there is a genetic defect in intestinal absorption, all cellular reactions which depend on that vitamin would be impaired. By contrast, if a vitamin is used by the cell in more than one way or in more than one coenzyme, a genetic abnormality might impair only a single reaction, leaving all others intact. Finally, abnormalities of specific apoprotein would be biochemically distinct and would leave other reactions catalyzed by the same vitamin intact. Thus one could expect symptoms ranging from those of the full-blown vitamin deficiency to a picture very different from that which occurs when the vitamin is not ingested. If the mutation involves a protein concerned with the metabolism of a particular vitamin, then no amount of the vitamin should correct the defect unless the block is circumvented by a different route of administration or unless the mutation is "leaky" (incomplete), leaving some residual activity which by the laws of mass action can be enhanced by supraphysiologic doses of the vitamin. Examples of all of these types of genetic diseases of vitamin metabolism have now been reported and are listed in Table 1.

The common features are early onset of life-threatening symptoms and signs, a dramatic response to supraphysiologic amounts of a single vitamin, and evidence for Mendelian inheritance implying the involvement of mutations at a single genetic locus.

As can be seen from Table 1, one or more of these abnormalities can be described with six different vitamins. The largest number of disorders described to date are those involving pyridoxine (B_6) responsiveness. In each of these the defect involves a single B_6-dependent apoenzyme such that cofactor supplementation restores enzymatic activity at least towards normal. The second group of disorders involves responsiveness to vitamin B_{12}, and these in some instances are due to defective vitamin metabolism and in others are due to defects in specific apoenzymes which require B_{12} as a cofactor. All of the disorders listed are rare. All, except B_6-responsive hypochromic anemia, appear to be inherited as an autosomal recessive. Nearly all of these conditions occur in infants or children, many in the neonatal period.

Three major clinical phenotypes have emerged in children with these vitamin-responsive genetic diseases. More than half of these disorders alter central nervous system development, leading to seizures, ataxia, mental retardation, or behavioral abnormalities. Hence, neonates or young infants with major neurologic disorders of ill-defined etiology must at least be considered candidates for a vitamin-responsive disorder. An almost equal number present with metabolic acidosis or ketosis and therefore any infant with unexplained disturbances in acid-base balance is a potential candidate for a vitamin-responsive disease. Finally, several conditions listed manifest anemia as a major presenting sign. Hence unexplained anemia should make the clinician think about certain vitamin-responsive diseases.

Table 1. Vitamin-responsive inherited metabolic diseases

Thiamin (vitamin B_1)
  Branched-chain ketoaciduria
  Cerebellar ataxia
  Lacticacidosis
  Megaloblastic anemia
Pyridoxine (vitamin B_6)
  Cystathioninuria
  Homocystinuria
  Hypochromic anemia
  Infantile convulsions
  Oxalosis
  Xanthurenic aciduria
Cobalamin (vitamin B_{12})
  Ileal transport defect
  Inert intrinsic factor
  Intrinsic factor deficiency
  Methylmalonicaciduria
  Methylmalonicaciduria and
    homocystinuria
  Transcobalamin II deficiency
Folic acid
  Formiminotransferase deficiency
  Homocystinuria and hypometh-
    ioninemia
  Intestinal malabsorption
  Megaloblastic anemia
Biotin
  β-Methylcrotonylglycinuria
  Propionicacidemia
Nicotinamide
  Hartnup disease
Vitamin D
  Familial rickets (autosomal)
  Familial rickets (X-linked)

The specific diagnosis of one of these disorders often involves specialized metabolic and diagnostic tests and is beyond the scope of this chapter. However, the alert physician, recognizing the signs and symptoms described above and unable to explain them, can perform a lifesaving function by referring such a child to a center that performs these tests. In a situation where this is impossible, empiric treatment with very large doses of the appropriate vitamin can be undertaken to see if the symptoms can be reversed.

RECOMMENDED READING

General

Kutsky, R. J., *Handbook of Vitamins and Hormones,* Van Nostrand Reinhold, New York, 1973.

Wagner, A. D., and K. Folkers, *Vitamins and Coenzymes,* Interscience, New York, 1964.

Biotin

McCormick, D. B., Biotin, *Nutr. Rev.,* **33**, 97 (1975).

Folic Acid

Bernstein, L. H., The Absorption and Malabsorption of Folic Acid and Its Polyglutamates, *Am. J. Med.,* **48**, 570 (1970).

Lindenbaum, J., Malabsorption in Vitamin B_{12} and Folate, in *Nutrition and Gastroenterology,* M. Winick, Ed., Wiley, New York (In press).

Roe, D., Nutrition and the Contraceptive Pill, in *Nutritional Disorders in American Women,* M. Winick, Ed., Wiley, New York, 1977, pp. 37–49.

Streiff, R. R., Folate Deficiency and Oral Contraceptives, *JAMA,* **214**, 105 (1970).

Niacin

Dietrich, L. S., Regulation of Nicotinamide Metabolism, *Am. J. Clin. Nutr.,* **24**, 800 (1971).

Nakagawa, I., T. Takahashi, A. Sasaki, M. Kajimoto, and T. Suzuki, Efficiency of Conversion of Tryptophan to Niacin in Humans, *J. Nutr.,* **103**, 1195 (1973).

Roe, D. A., *A Plague of Corn. The Social History of Pellagra.* Cornell University Press, Ithaca, 1973.

Pyridoxine (B_6)

Cinnamon, A. D., and J. R. Beaton, Biochemical Assessment of Vitamin B_6 Status in Man, *Am. J. Clin. Nutr.,* **23**, 696 (1970).

Committee on Nutrition, American Association of Pediatrics, Vitamin B_6 Requirements in Man, *Pediatrics*, **38**, 75 (1966).

Linkswiler, H., Biochemical and Physiologic Changes in Vitamin B_6 Deficiency, *Am. J. Clin. Nutr.*, **20**, 547 (1967).

Mudd, S. H., Pyridoxine-Responsive Genetic Disease, *Fed. Proc.*, **30**, 970 (1971).

Nelson, E. M., Association of Vitamin B_6 Deficiency with Convulsions in Infants, *Public Health Rep.*, **71**, 445 (1956).

Rose, D. P., R. Strong, J. Folkard, and P. W. Adams, Erythrocyte Aminotransferase Activities in Women Using Oral Contraceptives and the Effect of Vitamin B_6 Supplementation, *Am. J. Clin. Nutr.*, **26**, 48 (1973).

Rosenberg, L. E., Use of Cofactors in Inborn Errors of Amino Acid Metabolism, in *Nutritional Management of Genetic Disorders*, M. Winick, Ed., Wiley, New York, 1979, pp. 55–64.

Riboflavin

Horwitt, M. K., Nutritional Requirements of Man, with Special Reference to Riboflavin, *Am. J. Clin Nutr.*, **18**, 458 (1966).

McCormick, D. B., The Fate of Riboflavin in the Mammal, *Nutr. Rev.*, **30**, 75 (1972).

Rivlin, R. S., Riboflavin Metabolism, *N. Engl. J. Med.*, **13**, 626 (1970).

Rivlin, R. S., Ed., *Riboflavin*, Plenum, New York, 1975.

Thiamine

Sebrell, W. H., A Clinical Evaluation of Thiamine Deficiency, *Ann. New York Acad. Sci.*, **98,** 563 (1962).

Ziporin, Z. Z., W. T. Nunes, R. C. Powell, P. P. Waring, and H. E. Sauberlich, Thiamine Requirement in the Adult Human as Measured by Urinary Excretion of Thiamine Metabolites, *J. Nutr.*, **85,** 297 (1965).

Vitamin B_{12}

Herbert, V., Nutritional Requirements for Vitamin B_{12} Absorption and Folic Acid, *Am. J. Clin. Nutr.*, **21,** 743 (1968).

Maugh, T. H., Vitamin B_{12}, After 25 Years, the First Synthesis, *Science,* **179**, 266 (1973).

Stadtman, T. C., Vitamin B_{12}, *Science,* **171**, 859 (1971).

Toskes, P. P., and J. J. Deren, Vitamin B_{12} Absorption and Malabsorption, *Gastroenterology,* **65**, 662 (1973).

Vitamin C

Hodges, R. E., J. Hood, J. E. Canham, H. E. Sauberlich, and E. M. Baker, Clinical Manifestations of Ascorbic Acid Deficiency in Man, *Am. J. Clin. Nutr.*, **24,** 423 (1971).

King, C. G., Present Knowledge of Ascorbic Acid, *Nutr. Rev.*, **26**, 33 (1968).

Sherloch, P., and E. E. Rothchild, Scurvy Produced by a Zen Macrobiotic Diet, *JAMA,* **199**, 794 (1967).

10

MINERAL DEFICIENCIES

Deficiencies of a number of minerals can be produced in experimental animals and, in some cases, in humans. Most of these deficiencies occur in humans only in conjunction with another disease process and are rarely due to inadequate intake of the mineral alone. The major exceptions to this rule, and hence the minerals of most nutritional significance, are iron, calcium, and zinc. These three minerals may be ingested in inadequate amounts by significant numbers of people and hence primary deficiencies of these minerals occur with some frequency and may be corrected entirely by dietary means. Therefore, this chapter will deal primarily with these three minerals. The clinical consequences of other mineral deficiencies, such as magnesium, sodium and potassium, copper, selenium, chromium, and fluoride will be mentioned briefly.

IRON DEFICIENCY

The average healthy adult has about 4 g of total iron in his or her body. Hemoglobin accounts for about 2.5 g, tissue iron (myoglobin and cytochrome) about 0.3 g, and iron stores about 1 g. Iron is an essential component of three different processes involved in oxygen transfer. The body, therefore, has developed mechanisms to conserve and store iron. The normal daily losses in bile, feces, and sweat are small, and urinary excretion amounts to only about 1% of intake. In addition, in a healthy person iron is stored in the tissues bound to protein in a form known as ferritin.

Women during reproductive life lose additional iron as a result of menstruation. In some cases this may increase their requirement by as much as 1.5 mg/day. During the second and third trimesters of pregnancy the increasing red cell mass and fetal requirements together amount to 3 to 4 mg/day of iron. The total cost of pregnancy has been estimated at about 700 mg. In addition, there may be a large loss of hemoglobin due to hemorrhage during labor.

Growth imposes additional iron requirements. Fortunately, the healthy full-term infant is born with excess red cells which are temporarily converted into iron stores, but these are usually exhausted by the third or fourth month. The premature infant or the full-term infant with any of a variety of difficulties will not have this red cell excess and may even have a reduced number of red cells. Iron will therefore not be stored and the 3 to 4 month "grace" period will not exist.

After this variable period of time the requirements for growth must be met entirely by diet. During the first year this amounts to about 0.5 mg/day, decreasing during later childhood to 0.2 mg/day, and rising again during adolescence to 0.5 to 1.0 mg/day. One must also include in iron requirements the occasional bleeding which all individuals experience (0.5 mg of iron per ml of blood loss). Hence a blood donation of 450 ml, prorated over an entire year, will amount to 0.6 mg/day of iron, and increases the iron requirement in the adult male by 60%.

Body iron is maintained by a balance between iron intake, internal iron metabolism and redistribution, and iron loss. Figure 1 is a schematic representation of iron metabolism in man.

In all countries of the world people who eat a reasonably good diet obtain at least 12 mg/day of iron. However, the form that this iron takes in food is extremely important. Basically dietary iron is available in two forms: heme iron and nonheme or ionic iron. Heme iron is bound to porphyrin in hemoglobin and myoglobin. Absorption of heme iron is not affected by other dietary components and hence iron in this form is highly available (up to 35% in the iron-deficient subject). The heme complex is absorbed intact into the intestinal epithelial cell and only then is the iron split off. Nonheme iron is present in foods mainly as ferric hydroxide complexes, directly bound to organic molecules such as proteins, amino acids, and organic acids. Before such iron can be absorbed, it must be split from its complex and reduced to the divalent (ferrous) state. A number of components of the diet may affect this process and make the iron more or less available. For example, iron forms insoluble salts with phytates and phosphates in coarse vegetable foods. Such foods as corn, which is high in phytates, and egg yolks, which are high in phosphates, may not be as good sources of available iron as their actual iron content would suggest. Reducing substances, such as ascorbic acid, favor the absorption of ionic iron. Ascorbic acid promotes the reduction of ferric iron to the ferrous

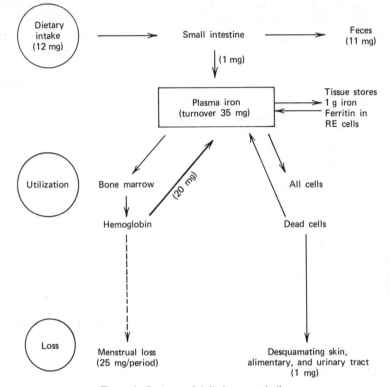

Figure 1. Pathway of daily iron metabolism.

form and also combines with iron to form a soluble chelate at a low pH. Meat releases the absorption of iron from other sources. Table 1 shows the percentage of iron absorbed from various common foods of vegetable and animal origin.

Hence both the quantity of iron present in food and the nature of that iron will determine how much is available for intake into the body. The point of regulation is iron absorption, which is influenced not only by the form of the iron in the diet, but also by the state of the iron reserves within the body.

Iron absorption does not occur in the stomach but takes place in the duodenum and upper small intestine. Gastric acid, however, plays a role in reducing ferric iron to ferrous iron, thereby rendering it more absorbable. In the intestinal mucosal cells, the iron may be either bound to the globulin transferrin and absorbed into the blood stream or combined with another protein, apoferritin, and deposited as ferritin within the mucosal cell itself, later to be lost as the cell is exfoliated.

what about the role of citrate?

Table 1. Iron absorption from food

Food	% of Iron Absorbed
Vegetable	Below 10
Rice	1
Spinach	1.5
Black beans	2.5
Corn	3.0
Lettuce	3.5
Wheat	5
Soya beans	6
Meat	Above 10
Veal liver	12–18
Fish muscle	10
Veal muscle	18–20
molasses	?

The two most important internal factors regulating iron absorption are (1) the state of iron stores, and (2) the state of activity of the bone marrow. When stores are low and new red cells are being rapidly produced, iron absorption is increased. This state is seen in growing children and in pregnant women. Absorption is also increased in anemia following hemorrhage or in anemia due to dietary iron deficiency. Neither the nature of the signals to the small intestine from the bone marrow and iron stores nor the control system within the intestinal wall which regulates the absorption of iron is fully understood. However, there is a suggestion that the concentration of transferrin iron within the cell may regulate the amount of iron absorbed by the cell.

Most body iron is present in circulating red cells. Since the life span of the erythrocyte is 120 days, 20 mg/day of iron is liberated in the adult male from catabolized red cells and assimilated by the erythron marrow into new erythrocytes. Total iron turnover is about 35 mg/day. Eighty percent of the total transferrin-bound iron is incorporated into erythrocytes. Each molecule of the iron-binding protein, transferrin, carries two molecules of iron. This protein releases iron selectively to tissues with high requirements, such as marrow or placenta. Normal transferrin-binding capacity is about 33 μg/100 ml of plasma and plasma iron is about 100 μg/100 ml of plasma. A useful index of iron status is transferrin saturation (plasma iron divided by iron-binding capacity) which is normally around 33% $\pm$ 15%. When this falls to 15% or less, insufficient iron is available to support normal hemoglobin formation.

Iron stores differ from country to country and from person to person. Average stores in adult male Americans are about 1000 mg, while in females about 300 mg are stored. The amount of circulating ferritin reflects the amount of stored iron, and recently methods have become available to determine serum ferritin.

As deficiency occurs the iron status of the body goes through a series of progressive changes. First serum ferritin falls, reflecting depletion of stores. This fall is accompanied by increased iron absorption followed by an increased iron-binding capacity of the plasma even though serum iron remains relatively normal. Following this stage, plasma iron falls and erythropoiesis is impaired. Red cell protoporphyrin increases from the normal 35 μg to over 100 μg/100 ml of red cells. Only in the final stage of depletion does the characteristic microcytic hypochromic anemia of iron deficiency occur accompanied by a fall in hemoglobin concentration.

Iron deficiency anemia is perhaps the most common nutritional deficiency disease in the United States. The ten state survey conducted by the Department of Health, Education, and Welfare in 1967 showed a high incidence of anemia in all age groups and in both sexes, particularly among our poorer populations. Certain populations are particularly vulnerable. Young infants who are not breast fed should be supplemented either by feeding an iron-containing formula or by giving supplemental iron in the form of drops. Children need to be encouraged to eat iron-rich foods. During adolescence this is particularly important, since both boys and girls will deplete iron stores during this period. Women during the reproductive age should also consume diets relatively rich in iron. During pregnancy, because of the marginal nature of the iron supply in our diets and because many women may have low stores at the outset, iron supplementation is recommended. This is particularly important in the pregnant teenager.

Although the symptoms of iron deficiency, even if moderate anemia is present, are nonspecific, recent evidence suggests that they are not without danger. For example, mildly anemic children did not perform as well in schools as similar children with normal levels of hemoglobin. Moreover, administration of iron rapidly improved school performance. In addition, hemoglobin concentration in older children has been used successfully as a screening method for picking up other nutritional deficiencies both in the child himself and in siblings. Thus it is incumbent on the physician not only to treat iron deficiency but to screen the entire family for iron deficiency and other nutritional deficiencies.

Severe iron deficiency in the adult is usually due to blood loss and its presence calls for a careful search for local disease of the gastrointestinal tract in the male and of the genital tract in the female. In children even severe deficiency (hemoglobins of 5 g or less) may be due to nutritional inadequacy. Treatment is iron replacement, and except under unusual circumstances the oral route is preferred.

CALCIUM DEFICIENCY

Calcium, which is the fifth most abundant element and the most abundant cation in the human body, comprises 1.5 to 2.0% of the total weight. More than 99% of calcium is present in bone in a ratio of 2:1 with phosphorus. Besides being the major support organ in the body, bone is an important physiologic tissue and is essential for maintenance of normal calcium balance. Bone is constantly formed and resorbed throughout life. As aging progresses, resorption predominates and there is a net bone loss. Although after the fifth decade this occurs in both men and women, it begins earlier in women and proceeds twice as rapidly until menopause.

The 1% of the body's calcium not present in bone is necessary for a number of essential functions and is found in extracellular fluid, soft tissue, and as a component of cell membranes. Calcium is involved in blood coagulation and is necessary for muscle contractility, for myocardial function, for normal neuromuscular irritability, and for maintaining the integrity of intracellular cement substances and various cell membranes. The activity of certain enzymes is also activated by calcium.

Serum calcium levels remain remarkably constant at a concentration of about 10 mg/100 ml. Decreases in serum calcium result in increased secretion of parathyroid hormone (PTH), which in turn stimulates the production of 1,25-dihydroxyvitamin D_3, resulting in increased intestinal absorption of calcium as well as increased resorption of calcium from bone. By contrast, increased levels of serum calcium reduce PTH secretion and increase calcitonin release. The production of 1,25-dihydroxyvitamin D_3 is reduced, resulting in reduced calcium absorption and reduced bone resorption.

Sixty percent of serum calcium is ionized and physiologically active. A significant decrease in serum ionized calcium results in tetany, while an increase can cause cardiac or respiratory failure.

Calcium is absorbed in the intestine by an active transport mechanism which depends on vitamin D. Phytates and oxalates in the diet decrease calcium absorption, whereas certain amino acids and lactose may enhance absorption. Two other dietary components play an important role in maintaining over-all calcium homeostasis: protein and phosphorus.

There is a definite relationship between dietary protein intake and calcium absorption and retention. At low protein intakes urinary calcium is low and calcium balance is positive even on intakes of 500 mg/day. Raising the protein level in the diet markedly increases calcium excretion in the urine. Although calcium absorption improves somewhat at higher protein levels patients with intakes of 100 g or more of protein were always in negative calcium balance. The improved absorption occurs as protein is raised from 50 to 100 g/day and when calcium intakes are 800 to 1400 mg/day. However, protein intakes above 100 mg/day do not increase absorption further. By contrast, urinary excretion of calcium increases as protein increases no matter what the dietary level of either protein or calcium. Thus, if the effect of protein intake on calcium absorption is limited while the effect on urinary calcium is unlimited, it becomes obvious that high intakes of protein adversely affect calcium nutrition at least in the adult. It should be noted that many Americans consume diets high in protein (100g/day or more) and relatively low in calcium (500 mg/day or less). Such a diet produced an average negative balance of 58 mg/day of calcium. This equals 21 g of calcium per year or 210 g in 10 years, more than 10% of the total body calcium.

The second important dietary constituent involved in calcium homeostasis is phosphorus. What seems to be critical is the Ca:P ratio in the diet. Ca:P ratios lower than 2:1 enhance bone resorption regardless of the absolute amount of calcium in the diet. Dietary phosphorus in many human diets is two to four times the calcium content, depending on the nature of the food supply. Diets high in meat, for example, would be expected to exert a negative effect on calcium balance both because of the high protein and because of the high phosphorus content.

From the above discussion it should be obvious that setting dietary requirements for calcium is at best extremely difficult. Realistic requirements can be set only in relation to protein intake and phosphorus intake. Moreover, if the intake of these nutrients is too high, negative calcium balance will result even at high calcium intakes. Thus the RDA for calcium, 800 mg/day in an individual consuming the average American diet, is at best a guess and may be misleading. To achieve an adequate net intake of calcium more attention should be paid to protein and phosphorus than to calcium itself.

Osteoporosis, a loss of calcium from bone, is estimated to cause sufficient bone loss to produce disabling symptoms in 14 million Americans. At present there is no evidence that high calcium intake will cure the disease, and the evidence that prolonged increase in calcium intake will prevent or delay the disease is tenuous. However, the recent data cited above, that the American diet because of its high protein and phosphorus content may be promoting negative calcium balance even at relatively high calcium intakes, makes one wonder whether osteoporosis may be at least in part a disease of nutritional origin.

There are some data which suggest that alveolar bone changes in the mandible associated with early periodontal disease may be reversed by the administration of 1 g of calcium daily for 1 year. It has been suggested that in some cases these changes may be the first signs of early osteoporosis.

Thus it is clear that calcium is required for the formation and maintenance of skeletal bone but the amount of calcium necessary under various dietary conditions remains unknown. The confusion is probably due to the multitude of factors, such as protein, phosphorus, fluoride, and hormonal factors, which influence calcium metabolism and bone mineralization. The RDA (800 mg/day) is probably reasonable under prevailing dietary conditions, although many people might benefit from somewhat higher intakes. Protein content and phosphorus content of the diet should be reduced if calcium retention is to be increased.

ZINC DEFICIENCY

Primary zinc deficiency has been recognized in man only recently, but evidence suggests that it might be a common mineral deficiency. Zinc is important in metabolism because it is an essential component of a number of enzyme systems and because of its influence on the structural configuration of certain nonenzyme organic ligands. Enzymes such as alkaline phosphatase, alcohol dehydrogenase, carbonic anhydrase, and lactic dehydrogenase, as well as a number of enzymes involved in nucleic acid metabolism, are zinc dependent. Some nonenzyme ligands with which zinc forms complexes are a macroglobulin glycoprotein in plasma, which firmly binds 30% of plasma zinc, and albumin, which loosely binds 65% of plasma zinc. Zinc can also bind to amino acids, transferrin, and nucleoproteins.

Because of its important role in many aspects of metabolism, many systems may be adversely affected by zinc deficiency, particularly if the deficiency occurs when cells of the particular system are rapidly dividing, growing, or synthesizing proteins. For example, gonadal maturation is severely retarded both in animals and in humans when dietary zinc is insufficient. During pregnancy, zinc deficiency in rats results in a high incidence of malformed and growth retarded offspring. In humans there has been a report that fetal size correlated directly with zinc concentration in amniotic fluid, and there has been speculation that the high incidence of congenital malformations in certain developing countries is due to habitual consumption of diets low in zinc. In addition, evidence suggests that cell mediated immunity may be adversely affected by zinc deficiency. Finally, zinc deficiency impairs normal tasting ability both in animals and in humans.

Primary zinc deficiency was first described in adolescent males from the Nile delta of Egypt. These children exhibited growth failure and hypogonadism. Subsequent studies confirmed the syndrome in girls and in younger children who displayed zinc-responsive growth failure and delayed sexual maturation. The primary cause of the syndrome appears to be the consumption of diets high in cereals. The phytates and fiber in the diets apparently inhibit the intestinal absorption of zinc by forming insoluble chelates. More recently, primary deficiency has been reported in people maintained on long-term parenteral nutrition (Chapter 22). Zinc analysis of the diets of some American children has revealed that zinc intakes are marginal. Similar findings have also been reported in American women. Plasma zinc levels normally decrease during pregnancy but the significance of this decrease is not known.

Secondary zinc deficiency can occur in alcoholism, chronic renal disease, hemolytic anemias, malabsorption syndromes, and patients suffering from severe trauma.

Although the exact requirement for zinc is not known, most diets contain from 10 to 15 mg/day, which is certainly adequate, Zinc is present in all meats, whole grain cereals, and legumes, but fruits and leafy vegetables are poor sources.

MAGNESIUM DEFICIENCY

Primary magnesium deficiency due to inadequate intake does not occur to our knowledge. However, secondary deficiency may accompany severe malabsorption, chronic alcoholism with malnutrition, parenteral nutrition with magnesium-free solutions coupled with large fluid losses from the gastrointestinal tract, large lactational losses in a previously nutritionally depleted woman, severe protein-calorie malnutrition in children, postnatal tetany syndromes, acute or chronic renal tubular disease, hypoparathyroidism, especially immediately after parathyroidectomy, and certain genetic disorders.

The signs and symptoms of magnesium deficiency in man relate to abnormalities in the metabolism of other minerals, namely, calcium and potassium. Thus magnesium deficiency results in faulty mobilization of calcium from bone, hypocalcemia, and hypokalemia. Hypocalcemia may result in tetany, hypokalemia in cardiac arrhythmias and even cardiac arrest. The low serum calcium and potassium will both respond to the administration of magnesium. By contrast, calcium administration will not reverse the hypocalcemia. In addition, magnesium deficiency results in certain neurological manifestations, presumably by direct effects of the deficiency on the central nervous system. These include personality changes, spontaneous generalized muscle spasms, tremor, fasciculations, and Trousseau and Chvostek signs. In some cases myoclonic jerks, athetoid movements, convulsions, and coma have been reported.

Clinically, it is important to remember that in any patient with low serum calcium or potassium, especially one who does not respond to the administration of these elements, magnesium deficiency should be suspected. Since low levels of serum magnesium may occur only after the patient is seriously depleted a trial of magnesium therapy is warranted even if serum magnesium levels are normal.

COPPER DEFICIENCY

It has been known for some time that copper, as well as iron, is required to prevent anemia in mammals maintained for long periods of time on cow's milk as the sole nutritional source. Normally the newborn liver stores enough copper to prevent deficiency during the nursing period. Hence primary copper deficiency is quite rare. However, secondary deficiency occurs in certain genetic diseases and in malabsorptive states associated with hypoproteinemia.

There are two well-defined genetic diseases in which copper metabolism is abnormal and serum copper levels are low in spite of an adequate dietary intake: Menkes' syndrome and Wilson's disease. Menkes' syndrome is a sex linked disease in the human male characterized by pili torti (kinky or steely hair), growth failure, cerebral degeneration, and early death. The pathology is similar to changes observed in copper-deficient animals. Copper concentrations in serum, liver, and brain are reduced. The basic defect is a failure to transport copper across membranes. Wilson's disease, or hepatolenticular degeneration, although it is also characterized by low serum copper levels, is associated with high levels of copper in tissues such as brain, liver, kidney, and cornea. Patients with this disease manifest cirrhosis and corneal degeneration. This, then, is not a nutritional deficiency even though serum copper levels are low. Treatment involves the use of chelating agents such as penicillamine to remove the excess copper, especially from the central nervous system.

Recently, copper deficiency has been described in severely malnourished children with histories of chronic diarrhea. These children, when treated with modified cow's milk, developed anemia, neutropenia, and bone demineralization, which failed to respond to iron but responded dramatically to the administration of oral copper. The sequence of events was: a drop in the level of serum copper and ceruloplasm, failure of iron absorption, neutropenia, leukopenia, bone demineralization, failure of erythropoiesis, and finally death. From this study it is important to remember that in a chronically malnourished patient with unexplained anemia that does not respond to conventional therapy the diagnosis of copper deficiency should be entertained and oral copper therapy instituted.

SELENIUM DEFICIENCY (KESHAN DISEASE)

In 1935, a disease of unknown etiology was reported from an area of China known as Keshan. The major clinical manifestations of the disease were acute signs of myocardial decompensation in young children and women in the childbearing age. Clinically the patients developed arrhythmias, cardiac failure with evidence of cardiomegaly on X-ray, and electrocardiographic changes indicative of myocardial damage. More careful observations determined that the disease occurred in a beltlike regional distribution extending from the northeast to the southwest of China. Large numbers of children and young adults were affected and in certain regions the mortality rate was well above 50%. Postmortem examination revealed extensive myocardial necrosis[6](Figure 2).

With the discovery of selenium deficiency in animals in the United States, it was noted that "white muscle disease" in cattle, a major manifestation of this deficiency, was prevalent in the same regional belt as Keshan disease. Moreover, analysis of foods raised in this region demonstrated low selenium levels. For these reasons, about 10 years ago a systematic investigation was undertaken by a specially created research unit of the Chinese Academy of Medical Sciences. Their epidemiological studies revealed that the disease was invariably associated with reduced levels of selenium in both serum and hair. In affected areas hair levels were below 0.12 PPM while in areas that were disease free levels exceeded 0.2 PPM. Both selenium loading tests and analysis of whole blood for glutathione peroxidase activity confirmed the marked selenium depletion of the population in the affected area.

Based on these results, a controlled intervention study, using sodium selenite (0.5 mg in 1 to 5 year olds and 1.0 mg in 6 to 9 year olds) was undertaken among children in Mianning County, Sichuan Province, from 1974 to 1977 inclusive. The incidence of Keshan disease in the supplemented group was 2.2% in 1974 and 1.0% in 1975. Untreated children in the control group had an incidence of 13.5% and 9.5% in 1974 and

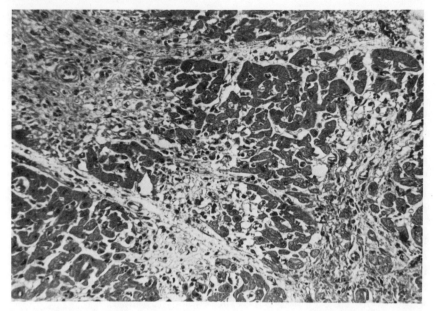

Figure 2. Pathological characteristics of Keshan disease (multiple focal myocardial necrosis with early fibrosis and slight cell infiltration). H.E. stain 200X. Courtesy of special Keshan Disease Unit, Beijing, China.

1975 respectively. (This was similar to the incidence of the disease in the 2 years prior to the intervention trial.) In addition, the disease was much less severe in the cases occurring in the treated group. For example, of 36,603 Se supplemented children, 21 cases of the disease occurred during the 4 years of investigation. Of these, only three died and one became chronic. Among 9642 children in the control group, 107 cases occurred, of which 53 died and six were in chronic heart failure.

Because of these results all children were treated in 1976 and 1977. The incidence of the disease dropped to 0.32% in 1976 and in 1977 there were no new cases. Thus supplementation of the population with sodium selenite effectively prevented the disease. At present, an attempt to fortify table salt with 15 PPM of sodium selenite is being tested, as is the efficacy of spraying crops in endemic areas with selenium. Initial results suggest that selenium content of grains can be increased by spraying. It should be noted that while selenium supplementation can effectively prevent the disease, it has no effect once the disease has occurred.

A number of observations suggest that selenium deficiency alone is not responsible for Keshan disease. First there is a direct seasonal incidence within the beltlike endemic area, winter in the north and summer in the south. Second, hair selenium levels were often equally low, within the endemic area, in individuals with or without Keshan disease. The Chinese investigating team currently believes that Keshan disease is due to selenium deficiency which creates conditions under which an acute environmental event, perhaps a viral infection, is likely to produce the myocardial damage. So far they have demonstrated viruslike inclusions in electron micrographs of myocardial tissue from patients who have died from Keshan disease, and they have isolated a strain of Coxsackie B virus from heart tissue of patients who died of the disease. Studies are in progress attempting to induce the disease in animals by producing a combination of selenium deficiency and viral infection.

Hence although the exact etiology of Keshan disease is still unknown, the disease can be effectively prevented by correcting the selenium deficiency. The unraveling of this disease is a clear demonstration by this Chinese research group of the importance of epidemiological observations coupled with carefully controlled intervention as a method for preventing a disease process even before the exact etiology is known.

OTHER MINERAL DEFICIENCIES

Cobalt is a constituent of vitamin B_{12} (cobalamin) and as such is essential. Since it must be consumed in the form of B_{12}, no other requirement for cobalt is necessary.

There is still considerable controversy over whether fluoride is an essential element. There is no doubt, however, that fluoride is concentrated in apatite, and is therefore present in greatest quantity in calcified tissues. In descending order the highest fluoride contents are found in cementum, bone, dentin, and enamel. Since higher fluoride content in tooth enamel renders the tooth more resistant to dental caries, fluoridation of drinking water has been recommended and adopted in many areas. At present it is believed that ingestion of 1 ppm/day of fluoride in temperate climates will produce a good anticariogenic effect while not causing teeth to have a brownish mottled appearance. It should be understood that while fluoride ingestion will help prevent caries, dental caries is not a fluoride deficiency disease but rather a complex multifactorial disease produced by bacteria using a sugar substrate (see Chapter 14). Thus under normal circumstances fluoride may not be essential, but as we shall discuss in the next section, changes in our lifestyle may be slowly converting a nonessential to an essential dietary component.

SUPPLEMENTAL VITAMINS AND MINERALS

Vitamins and certain minerals are essential nutrients necessary for life and maintenance of good health. They cannot be manufactured in sufficient amounts in the human body and therefore man must get them from his food supply. Both vitamins and minerals are widely spread through animal and plant species, making it possible to obtain them on a variety of diets and eating patterns. Certainly it is no surprise that in very poor people, who do not get enough to eat, vitamin and mineral deficiencies of various types are found. What is more surprising is that in the developed countries of the world, particularly in the United States, presumably the best fed country in the world, millions of people pop a vitamin pill into their mouths each morning. Is there any reason for this behavior? Or is this just one more manifestation of a "pill popping culture," a manifestation which has made human urine perhaps the richest natural source of vitamins on earth.

Certainly it would appear that we should be able to get all the vitamins and minerals we need from our abundant food supply, and yet when we examine the eating patterns and over-all lifestyles of most Americans one cannot be sure.

Let us begin with the propagation of the human species, pregnancy. During pregnancy, as we have seen, the requirements for vitamins and minerals increase, particularly those for folic acid, vitamin B_{12}, calcium, and iron. Presumably these requirements are to be met by the pregnant woman's increasing her over-all food intake, which would supply additional amounts of these and other nutrients. However, until quite recently, pregnant women have been advised to keep their weight gain down by limiting food intake. The result is that vitamin and mineral intake is limited; the solution—a multivitamin pill. Even now that the trend is being reversed and pregnant women are being allowed to eat more and gain more, the above nutrients remain in marginal supply and supplementation is recommended. Our current eating patterns and over-all lifestyles make availability of these nutrients at best marginal, especially in women.

The human infant, like all mammalian infants, was meant to be breast fed. The breast fed infant does not develop vitamin or mineral deficiencies, with the possible exception of vitamin D deficiency in infants completely shielded from sunlight. However, in our culture, only a minority of infants are breast fed. Originally, when formulas were prepared from cow's milk, water, and added sugar, vitamins A, C, and D, as well as iron, were supplemented in the form of drops. More recently, with the emergence of infant formulas, these nutrients have been added to the mixture. Thus, until recently, many if not most of our infants required vitamin and mineral supplementation even though breast milk contained all the vitamins and minerals they needed. There has been a tendency to introduce solid foods earlier and earlier, a tendency that has continued right up to the present. The young infant, sometimes 6 weeks old or less, is usually introduced to cereal, and as a justification for this totally unphysiologic situation iron has been added to the cereal. Again we are supplementing because we have created an eating pattern for the infant that now requires supplementation, a sort of nutritional "Catch 22." It is interesting to note that until recently most of the iron added to infant cereals was not absorbed because of the form it was in. This situation has now been corrected.

The practice of vitamin and mineral supplementation reached its peak in young children. It represented a sort of insurance policy against malnutrition and it relieved parents and physicians of the responsibility of learning about nutrition and foods. As Chapter 15 points out, the widespread fortification of many foods, especially with vitamin D, may lead to cumulative storage and ultimate toxicity. This is particularly true when vitamin supplements containing vitamin D are also used.

At present, especially since many foods are being fortified, I see little indication for vitamin and mineral supplementation in school age children who are eating a reasonably good diet.

The adolescent presents a problem in modern society because many have adopted bizarre eating habits. Again, if a reasonable diet is consumed, there is no indication for vitamin and mineral supplementation. However, many adolescents, even in affluent populations, have reduced levels of vitamins or minerals (especially iron). If the eating patterns of an adolescent preclude the ingestion of adequate amounts of vitamins and minerals, then supplementation with a multivitamin preparation and iron may be warranted. However, every attempt to change those eating patterns should be made first.

In the adult population, the decision whether certain individuals should be routinely supplemented is not an easy one. As has been pointed out, heavy alcohol consumption may adversely affect the metabolism of certain vitamins (thiamin and folate), and heavy smoking may reduce vitamin C levels. When these habits are added to the constant struggle for weight maintenance and the consumption of some of the fad diets of the day, intakes of certain vitamins and minerals are lower than they should be. In spite of this, there is little evidence that the average adult male has any signs of lowered vitamin or mineral levels, and hence I would not recommend routine supplementation in adult males. In the female the situation is different. In addition to the high incidence of heavy alcohol consumption and smoking, iron loss through menstruation, vitamin depletion during pregnancy and lactation (if supplementation has not been given), use of contraceptive pills (which interfere with folate and B_6 metabolism), and consumption of high protein, high phosphate diets (which promote negative calcium balance), are common in the female. Moreover the American woman is extremely weight conscious, and is often consuming a severely restricted diet. Millions of women (and men as well) are consuming drugs in the form of tranquilizers and other medications whose effects on vitamin and mineral metabolism are unknown.

Hence, the dilemma. Should we add another pill to the lifestyle of the average American woman? Should we try in some way to modify that lifestyle? Certainly we as physicians must take a little of the responsibility for the problem as it exists. Many busy physicians have certainly succumbed to the convenience of prescribing a pill. Now we are faced with the problem of perhaps having to give another.

My own position is that we as a profession should begin to resist the tendency for vitamin and mineral supplementation without indication. This means that we must take dietary histories, evaluate symptoms carefully, and sometimes determine blood values for certain vitamins and minerals. Certainly if a woman is deficient, specific therapy should be given. However, this therapy should be for a short time and the diet should be improved so that deficiency will not recur.

Older Americans form yet another population, the fastest growing population at present. Here, too, lifestyles may adversely affect proper vitamin and mineral intake. Older people often consume convenience foods, which may be low in certain vitamins and minerals. In addition, they are often living on low incomes, and hence may try to save by cutting out more expensive foods. Finally, they may have specific problems that affect vitamin or mineral metabolism. Many are completely or partially edentulous and hence must consume soft foods; most have some degree of gastric atrophy and achlorhydria, which can cause problems with iron and vitamin B_{12} absorption. There are no good nutritional surveys on the elderly in America (yet another indication of their neglect), and hence it is not possible to even estimate the extent of vitamin and mineral deficiency that exists in that population.

My own feeling at present is that until we can learn more, old people with any history of dietary inadequacies should be supplemented, especially with iron and vitamin B_{12}.

Before concluding, let me address an issue that will arise again when we discuss megavitamin therapy. Many people who advocate the routine use of vitamin supplementation argue that although it might not be necessary to prevent deficiency, it is necessary to "promote optimal health." The fact that some people claim to feel better when they take a vitamin tablet may or may not be significant. Certainly there is no objective evidence that individuals who are not vitamin depleted increase their general well being by consuming extra vitamins or minerals.

Another argument often used is that at least the water-soluble vitamins are not toxic and hence taking them just as insurance cannot hurt. Again I cannot accept this argument. We are learning more and more that toxicity may take years, in some cases almost a lifetime, to manifest itself. Thus although we know of no toxicity at present, we cannot rule out its potential. To me it is interesting that often the same people concerned with the long-term effects of sugar or fat in the diet or food additives or environmental pollutants show no concern about, and in fact advocate, the use of unphysiologic amounts of vitamins and minerals over an entire lifespan.

In summary, in a culture that consumes large amounts of alcohol, smokes vast numbers of cigarettes, takes millions and perhaps billions of contraceptive and other pills per year, in a culture that is constantly dieting because of previous overconsumption, at least the female population is at risk for certain vitamin and mineral deficiencies. The situation has progressed to the extent that during periods of particular stress, for example, pregnancy and lactation, supplementation is definitely indicated. At other times it is still possible to attemp dietary therapy, which will not only correct the deficiency but will also begin to make some progress in altering lifestyles. Time, however, may be running out and unless the trend is reversed, we may soon find ourselves in the position of having to give routine vitamin supplementation.

RECOMMENDED READING

Calcium

Alvarez, W. C., Osteoporosis, a Disease that Attacks Millions, *Geriatrics*, **25**, 77 (1970).

Coulston, A., and L. Lutwak, Dietary Calcium Deficiency and Human Peridontal Disease, *Fed. Proc.*, **31**, 721 (1972).

Gain, S. M., Adult Bone Loss, Fracture Epidemiology and Nutritional Implications, *Nutrition*, **27**, 107 (1973).

Lutwak, L., Nutritional Aspects of Osteoporosis, *J. Am. Geriat. Soc.*, **17**, 115 (1969).

Tanaka, Y., H. Frank, and H. F. De Luca, Intestinal Calcium Transport, Stimulation by Low Phosphorous Diet, *Science*, **181**, 564 (1973).

Walker, R. M., and H. M. Linkswiler, Calcium Retention in the Adult Human Male as Affected by Protein Intake, *J. Nutr.*, **102**, 1297 (1972).

Iron

Bothwell, T. H., and C. A. Finch, *Iron Metabolism*, Little, Brown, Boston, 1962.

Crosby, W. H., Intestinal Response to the Body's Requirement for Iron, Control of Iron Absorption, *JAMA*, **208**, 347 (1969).

Finch, C. A., Iron Deficiency Anemia, *Am. J. Clin. Nutr.*, **22**, 512 (1969).

Greenberger, N. J., Effects of Antibiotics and Other Agents on Intestinal Transport of Iron, *Am. J. Clin. Nutr.*, **26**, 104 (1973).

Katzman, R., A. Novack, and A. Pearson, Nutritional Anemia in an Inner-City Community. Relation to Ages and Ethnic Group, *JAMA*, **222**, 670 (1972).

Schaffrin, R. M., J. W. Thomas, and T. D. Stout, The Effects of Blood Donation on Serum Iron and Hemoglobin Levels in Young Women, *Canad. Med. A. J.*, **104**, 229 (1971).

Sturgeon, P., and A. Shoden, Total Liver Storage Iron in Normal Populations of the U.S.A., *Am. J. Clin. Nutr.*, **24**, 469 (1971).

Van Campen, D., Regulation of Iron Absorption, *Fed. Proc.*, **33**, 100 (1974).

Selenium

Keshan Disease Research Group of the Chinese Academy of Medical Sciences, Beijing, Epidemiologic Studies on the Etiologic Relationship of Selenium and Keshan Disease, *Chinese Med. J.*, **92**(7), 477–482 (1979).

Keshan Disease Research Group of the Chinese Academy of Medical Sciences, Beijing, Observations on Effect of Sodium Selenite in Prevention of Keshan Disease, *Chinese Med. J.*, **92**(7), 471–476 (1979).

Scott, M. L., The Selenium Dilemma, *J. Nutr.*, **103,** 803 (1973).

Stadtman, T. C., Selenium Biochemistry, *Science*. **183,** 915 (1974).

Zinc

Food and Nutrition Board, Zinc in Human Nutrition, N.R.C., Washington, D.C. (1970).

Prasad, A. S., *Zinc Metabolism*. Thomas, Springfield, Ill., 1966.

Sanstead, H. H., Zinc Nutrition in the United States, *Am. J. Clin. Nutr.*, **26**, 1251 (1973).

Other Minerals

Gedalia, I., and I. Zipkin, *The Role of Fluoride in Bone Structure*, Green, St. Louis, 1973.

Hambridge, K. M., Chromium Nutrition in Man, *Am. J. Clin. Nutr.*, **27**, 505 (1974).

Mertz, W., Recommended Dietary Allowances up to Date—Trace Minerals, *J. Am. Dietet. Assoc.*, **64**, 163 (1974).

Mertz, W., and W. E. Cornatzer, *Newer Trace Elements in Nutrition*. Marcel Dekker, New York, 1971.

Nielson, F. H., "Newer" Trace Elements in Human Nutrition, *Food Tech.*, **28**, 38 (1974).

Nielson, F. H., and H. H. Sanstead, Are Nickel, Vanadium, Silicon, Fluoride and Tin Essential for Man? *Am. J. Clin. Nutr.*, **27**, 515 (1974).

Underwood, E. J., Cobalt, *Nutr. Rev.*, **33**, 65 (1975).

11
DEFICIENCY OF DIETARY FIBER

One major change in lifestyle connected with our western way of living has been a reduction in the intake of fiber. The pipeline from food producer to food consumer has lengthened. The need for long-term storage of large quantities of food has resulted in a reduction of food bulk. Foods have become more and more refined and the natural fiber content in the foods we eat has declined. There is evidence that certain diseases that have been increasing in western society may be caused, at least in part, by our relatively low fiber diet.

When we talk about fiber, we are referring to the portion of our food that remains undigested and contributes little or no calories to our diet. For practical purposes we are talking about the bran supplied by a variety of cereal grains and the pectins and other fibers derived from fruit and vegetable sources. Much of this fiber, although not all, is complex polysaccharide material such as cellulose, hemicellulose, and others.

DISEASES ASSOCIATED WITH FIBER DEFICIENCY

In the past few years a great deal has been written about the importance of fiber in our diet and a number of diseases have been ascribed to a deficiency of dietary fiber. Some of the evidence for these claims is reasonably solid, whereas some is simply anecdotal. Table 1 lists those diseases most often mentioned as being related to fiber deficiency.

Table 1.   Digestive diseases and disorders attributed in part to deficiency of dietary vegetable fiber

---

Chronic constipation
Diverticular disease of the colon
Carcinoma of the colon
Cholelithiasis
Hiatus hernia
Hemorrhoids
Appendicitis

Chronic Constipation

Chronic constipation heads the list because it is so prevalent in our society, especially among the elderly, and because the evidence linking it with dietary fiber deficiency is strong. The disease, while certainly not life threatening, produces a great deal of discomfort. Epidemiologic data clearly demonstrate that the amount of fiber in the diet positively correlates with the size of the stools and that this amount of fiber is inversely related to the time required for the evacuation of residues. These correlations are attributed to cumulative absorption of fecal matter water with longer retention in the colon. Recently these epidemiologic studies have been confirmed by direct measurements of absorption of water from the intestinal lumen.

Many clinical reports, most of them without adequate controls, strongly indicate that restoration of the bulk of the stools by using bran or cellulose/hemicellulose preparations will significantly relieve chronic constipation. Stool weights have consistently shown an increase as a result of such treatment. Hence, in our society, the evidence suggests that although chronic constipation is undoubtedly related to many factors, a major contributor is the highly refined low fiber diet being consumed.

Diverticular Disease

Diverticular disease is a major and disabling problem and increases in frequency as the population ages. It is estimated that this disease affects between 5 and 10% of our population over 60 years of age. The prevalence of asymptomatic diverticuli is estimated to be four or five times as high. Table 2 indicates the prevalence of diverticulosis in the general population. Clearly this disease is age related. In addition, epidemiologic evidence

Table 2. Prevalence of diverticulosis in the general population (radiological survey)

Age	No. of Subjects	No. with Diverticula	Prevalence (%)
Under 40	39	0	0.0
40–59	27	5	18.5
60–79	24	7	29.2
Over 80	19	8	42.1

suggests that the disease is much more prevalent in western developed countries, and that differences between countries occur not on a racial basis but rather on an environmental basis. Japanese who migrate to Hawaii or California and who adopt a western style diet develop a pattern of frequent diverticuli similar to that of Americans. By contrast, those who retain Japanese eating habits will show the same low incidence as in Japan.

The low fiber hypothesis has been supported further by the experimental production of colonic diverticuli in aging laboratory animals consuming diets unnaturally low in fiber. The best hypothesis for explaining the mechanism by which this occurs is that the increased stool bulk which results from more dietary fiber will increase the diameter of the colon. It is well known that the pressure generated by any peristaltic contraction is inversely proportional to the diameter of the bowel. Thus the greater the bulk, the less the intraluminal pressure. Diverticuli are herniations of mucosa and submucosa of the colon through the circular muscular layer. They are actually propulsion diverticuli. The essential condition, aside from muscular defects in the intestinal wall, is increased intraluminal pressure.

There is good evidence that patients with diverticular disease have increased intraluminal pressure at rest and after bowel stimulation by either eating or neostigmine injection (Table 3). Moreover, in patients

Table 3. Sigmoid motility studies "total pressure"

	Normal	Diverticular Disease
Basal	10.77 ± 3.3	56.61 ± 10.6
After eating	31.57 ± 5.0	174.81 ± 25.3
Neostigmine	53.08 ± 10.6	177.87 ± 17.4

with diverticular disease this increased pressure can be reduced after feeding 20 g of bran daily for several weeks to several months (Table 4).

Clinical experience with the use of bran supplements in diverticular disease has been generally good although the number of controlled studies is again limited. It is extremely important for this point to be clarified as soon as possible because many physicians have been taught to treat diverticular disease with low residue, low fiber diets. This has come about largely because of the presence of fibers and seed in diverticuli and the conclusion that they might be causing the problem. Present evidence indicates that this is not so, and more and more experience is suggesting the ingestion of *increased* fiber in the treatment of diverticular disease and increased fiber in the general population for the prevention of diverticular disease.

Carcinoma of the Colon

Cancer of the colon (including the rectum) is the most common cancer of the digestive tract in the United States. It accounts for nearly 50,000 deaths per year, and is exceeded in this respect only by carcinoma of the lung. The epidemiologic data are similar to those of diverticulosis, suggesting environmental influences in western society. Moreover careful analysis of these data shows the strongest correlations between colon cancer and two dietary constituents—*total fat and animal protein.*

The bulk of evidence suggests that whereas excess fat and animal proteins in our diet are probably the most important dietary constituents in the pathogenesis of colon cancer, deficiency in dietary fiber probably also plays a role. At present, the best working hypothesis suggests that the fat and protein in the bowel allow for a bacterial flora which will break down these substances. Some of these breakdown products are precarcinogens. In addition, products of bile salt excretion into the gastrointestinal tract are also known to be potentially carcinogenic. Fiber plays two roles. First

Table 4. Sigmoid motility before and after methylcellulose treatment

	Colonic Motility Index		
	Before	After	P
Resting	7577	1236	<0.025
During feeding	13,592	2645	<0.01
Postprandial	8237	1761	<0.05

it binds bile acids, and second it decreases transit time and therefore decreases the amount of time the lumen is exposed to these potential cancer-producing agents.

The high incidence of cancer of the colon is undoubtedly due to a number of interacting dietary factors present in the typical western diet which result in an increased quantity of carcinogens and an increased time of exposure of the intestinal mucosa to these carcinogens. Low fiber content appears to be one of the dietary factors.

Cholelithiasis (Gallstones)

Present ideas about the formation of gallstones suggest that the problem arises because of an imbalance in the kind of bile acids secreted by the liver. Normally the balance between cholic and chenodeoxycholic acid is such that the amount of cholesterol in the bile is kept to a minimum. If too little "cheno" is present, cholesterol in bile becomes high and will deposit in stones.

Fiber deficiency in man leads to a reduced synthesis of bile salts and a decrease in their total concentration in bile. Feeding bran increases not only total bile salt content but also the relative "cheno" content. Thus bran fed in levels that can be supplied in the diet can correct abnormalities in biliary lipids which, if allowed to continue for prolonged periods, result in the formation of gallstones.

Other Diseases

At present there are few data indicating that any of the other diseases listed is caused by dietary fiber deficiency. In addition there are some data which suggest that the high incidence of stomach cancer in some countries may be due in part to the *high* dietary intake of fiber in those countries.

Two other diseases, not mentioned in the table, are currently being investigated in relation to dietary fiber deficiency—diabetes and arteriosclerosis.

Some data suggest that increasing the fiber content in the diet of diabetics may lower the blood sugar levels and even the insulin requirement. The mechanism that is postulated is a binding of sugar in the intestine which results in a slower rate of absorption. Studies in this area are extremely limited but the importance of the concept is such that it promises to be an active area for future investigations.

Conflicting data exist about the role of fiber in arteriosclerosis. Some studies suggest that high fiber diets will lower serum cholesterol and triglycerides. Other studies have failed to confirm these observations.

Again the importance of the problem is such that more studies will undoubtedly be done in the near future.

COMMENT

Keeping the data presented above in mind, how should patients be advised? Certainly I can see no real contraindications to increasing the fiber content of the American diet. Especially beginning in middle age, eating more salad, fruits, and vegetables is to be encouraged. In addition I see no reason not to encourage the use of bran in this period of life, especially if there is any history of constipation.

Although I am not sure how much protection will be offered from diverticulitis, cholelithiasis, and cancer of the colon, the incidence of these combined diseases, their combined mortality and morbidity, and the economic loss they generate is so staggering that any reduction in incidence would be important. In addition, it is possible that some benefit may accrue in reducing the incidence of coronary artery disease and in the management of diabetes.

RECOMMENDED READING

Albersheim, P., The Walls of Growing Plant Cells, *Scientific American,* **232**, 80, April (1975).

Almy, T. P., The Role of Fiber in the Diet, in *Nutrition and Aging,* M. Winick, Ed., Wiley, New York, 1976, pp. 155-69.

Cummings, J. H., Progress Report: Dietary Fiber, *Gut,* **14**, 69 (1973).

Dietary Fiber and Colonic Function—An Effect of Particle Size, *Nutr. Rev.,* **33**, 70 (1975).

Kritchevsky, D., and J. A. Story, Dietary Fiber and Cancer, in *Nutrition and Cancer.* M. Winick, Ed., Wiley, New York, 1979, pp. 41-54.

Painter, N. S., A. Z. Almeida, and K. W. Colebourne, Unprocessed Bran in Treatment of Diverticular Disease of the Colon, *Brit. Med. J.,* **2**, 137 (1972).

Payler, D. K., E. W. Pomare, K. W. Heaton, and R. F. Harvey, The Effect of Wheat Bran on Intestinal Transit, *Gut,* **16**, (1975).

PART III

NUTRIENT EXCESS

12

EXCESS CALORIES

OBESITY AS A PUBLIC HEALTH PROBLEM

Obesity may be the most serious health problem in America today. Ten to 13% of children are overweight and 80% of all overweight children become overweight adults. Obesity is associated with an increased risk of heart disease by increasing the chances of an individual's being hyperlipidemic or hypertensive. The higher prevalence of hypertension, in turn, increases the risk of cerebrovascular accidents. Obesity is also associated with an increased incidence of adult-onset diabetes and with all the complications that may follow. Thus obesity kills through its complications. It should be noted that people who are obese but who develop none of these complications do not have a reduced life expectancy. In fact, some data suggest that such people may actually live longer.

This concept that obesity kills through its complications is an important one when the public health consequences of this disease are examined. Obesity is more common in women than in men. It is particularly prevalent among poor black women. However, since the mortality from cardiovascular disease is much higher in men than in women, obesity may be a more serious disease in men. What is needed, and what has not been addressed by the medical profession, is the establishment of criteria for populations and individual patients who are at risk not only for obesity but for the complications of obesity.

In addition to an increased mortality and morbidity due to its complications, obesity itself leads to considerable inconvenience within our society. The obese person leads a more difficult life. Thin is the image that Americans have adopted as chic. The fat person is afflicted with many social problems even though 20% of the population is overweight. It has been said that the obese may one of the most oppressed minorities in America.

Thus for both medical and social reasons, obesity represents a challenge to the health professional, a challenge that until recently has not been seriously accepted.

DEFINITION

Obesity can be defined as a relative increase in total body fat. Thus at any given weight an individual can be obese if body fat makes up too much of total body mass. In adults, we have used weight for height as a reasonable estimate of total body fat. In children, weight for height corrected for age has been used. Table 1 gives the "ideal" weight for height for adult men and women. It should be remembered that while these are good approximations for average people, there are certain important exceptions. For example, the athlete who weighs 240 lb and is 6 ft 1 in. may not be obese. Much of the increased weight is due to an increase in lean body mass.

Recently, obesity has been defined at the cellular level, and by using this definition, we can distinguish at least two distinct forms of obesity. Many individuals, often those with mild or moderate obesity beginning in middle age, have an adipose tissue depot that is made up of a normal number of adipocytes each containing a very large fat droplet (type I, or hypertrophic obesity). Other individuals, often those with marked obesity and a history dating to early childhood, have an adipose depot made up of *too many* adipocytes each containing a fat droplet reasonably normal in size (type II, or hyperplastic obesity). Figure 1 diagrammatically represents these two conditions.

During weight reduction, only the size of the fat cell is reduced; the number of fat cells is not affected. Hence, an obese person whose fat cells are just too large can reduce the size of each fat cell to normal and will then have adipose tissue identical in every respect to that in thin persons (Figure 2, type I). By contrast, an obese individual who has too many fat cells that are normal in size will have to reduce the size of those fat cells to *below* normal in order to maintain a normal quantity of adipose tissue. This person will still have too many fat cells (Figure 2, type II) and will now be in the doubly abnormal state of having too many too small fat cells. These people have a particularly difficult time maintaining the reduced body weight.

The significance of the discovery of type II (hyperplastic) obesity is that preventive measures must be taken early in life if this type of obesity is to be avoided. The evidence suggests that there are two critical periods

Table 1. Desirable weight for men and women aged 25 and over[a] (in pounds according to height and frame, in indoor clothing)

Height[b]				
Feet	Inches	Small Frame	Medium Frame	Large Frame
		Men		
5	2	112–120	118–129	126–141
5	3	115–123	121–133	129–144
5	4	118–126	124–136	132–148
5	5	121–129	127–139	135–152
5	6	124–133	130–143	138–156
5	7	128–137	134–147	142–161
5	8	132–141	138–152	147–166
5	9	136–145	142–156	151–170
5	10	140–150	146–160	155–174
5	11	144–154	150–165	159–179
6	0	148–158	154–170	164–184
6	1	152–162	158–175	168–189
6	2	156–167	162–180	173–194
6	3	160–171	167–185	178–199
6	4	164–175	172–190	182–204
		Women		
4	10	92–98	96–107	104–119
4	11	94–101	98–110	106–122
5	0	96–104	101–113	109–125
5	1	99–107	104–116	112–128
5	2	102–110	107–119	115–131
5	3	105–113	110–122	118–134
5	4	108–116	113–126	121–138
5	5	111–119	116–130	125–142
5	6	114–123	120–135	129–146
5	7	118–127	124–139	133–150
5	8	122–131	128–143	137–154
5	9	126–135	132–147	141–158
5	10	130–140	136–151	145–163
5	11	134–144	140–155	149–168
6	0	138–148	144–159	153–173

[a] Prepared by Metropolitan Life Insurance Co.; data derived primarily from Build and Blood Pressure Study, 1959, Society of Actuaries.
[b] Height in shoes.

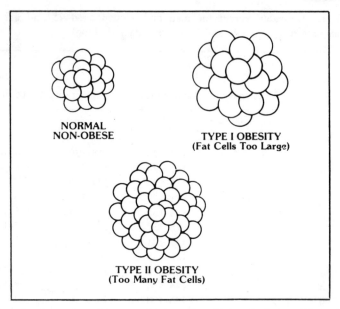

Figure 1. Comparison of hypertrophic (type I) and hyperplastic (type II) obesity.

in life when too many fat cells may develop—infancy and adolescence. Overfeeding during these critical periods may lead to a permanent abnormality with which a person must struggle throughout life—excessive numbers of fat cells.

ETIOLOGY

Recent evidence implies that obesity is a disease with multiple causes. Both genetics and environment contribute in determining the amount of body fat and the cellular makeup of the adipose depot. Animal experiments suggest that the rate of cell division within the adipose depot is to some extent under genetic control. Moreover, the cells within the adipose depot in certain genetically obese strains of rodents continue to divide long past the time when cell division has ceased in the adipose depot of lean littermates. Observations of identical human twins raised in completely different environments suggest that their body types, whether lean or fat, tend to be the same. By contrast, fraternal twins raised in different environments will tend to have different body types. Thus a certain amount of obesity has a genetic basis and no doubt this kind of obesity is more difficult to

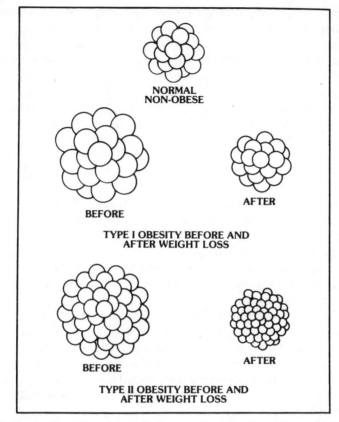

Figure 2. Result of weight reduction in hypertrophic (type I) and hyperplastic (type II) obesity.

control. The precise incidence of this type of obesity, its cellular makeup, and just how purely it occurs are still unknown.

By far the most common type of obesity is environmentally induced; that is, more calories are consumed than expended over a variable period of time. This type of obesity may begin in middle life when eating patterns have been established and exercise is replaced by martinis, or it may begin in early life when parents struggle to stuff their children in a well-meaning but misguided attempt to keep them healthy. The average American 6-month-old is consuming 135% of the recommended daily amount of calories. From whatever the original food source, excess calories will be converted to fat and deposited into the adipose depot. What makes the problem much more difficult, however, is that because of individual metabolic differences what is a slight excess for one individual may not be an excess for another. Minute differences in metabolic rate, in specific dynamic action, in "activity" at rest, and in energy expenditure during exercise, when sustained over long periods of time, can account for large differences in weight between two individuals who are consuming similar amounts of calories and expending what appears to be similar amounts of energy. The observation that one person will gain weight although he consumes fewer calories than another who gains none is no doubt valid.

DIAGNOSIS

The diagnosis of obesity can be made with different degrees of accuracy. Is the distribution of adipose tissue and lean body mass such that there is a relatively larger proportion of fat tissue? In most adults, simply comparing weight for height is enough. In children, weight for height corrected for age is often used. As pointed out above, this method is not always correct and is most inaccuracte for individuals who are only slightly obese, the very individual in whom the diagnosis may be most difficult to make. Recently, the use of skinfold calipers has become more prevalent in the diagnosis of obesity. With proper use of these instruments a precise diagnosis can usually be made. Recent evidence suggests that in experienced hands, measurement of triceps and subscapular fatfold thickness is as accurate a method for determining total body fat as the methods of determining total body water or potassium. Table 2 shows normal fatfold thicknesses for men and women.

Once obesity has been diagnosed, the type of obesity can be ascertained. While precise diagnosis of type I or type II obesity requires an adipose tissue biopsy, a good approximation can be obtained from the history. Although not all childhood obesity is hyperplastic, most individuals with hyperplastic obesity will have a history of obesity since childhood. Although not all severe obesity is hyperplastic, most individuals with hyperplastic obesity are severely obese. Hence, a severely obese individual with a clear history of obesity since childhood is potentially an individual with hyperplastic obesity.

The diagnosis of genetic obesity is at best very difficult and may not be possible except in extraordinary situations. We know that if one parent is obese there is a 40% chance that the child will be obese. If both parents are obese, the chance increases to 80%. We know that fat women are more likely to marry fat men and vice versa. Although this might suggest genetic influences that can be historically traced, environmental explanations may be equally applicable. Simply stated, obese parents may overfeed their

Table 2.   Triceps skinfold percentiles[a]

Age (Years)	Males Percentiles (mm)					Females Percentiles (mm)				
	5th	15th	50th	85th	95th	5th	15th	50th	85th	95th
Birth-	4	5	8	12	15	4	5	8	12	13
0.5-	5	7	9	13	15	6	7	9	12	15
1.5-	5	7	10	13	14	6	7	10	13	15
2.5-	6	7	9	12	14	6	7	10	12	14
3.5-	5	6	9	12	14	5	7	10	12	14
4.5-	5	6	8	12	16	6	7	10	13	16
5.5-	5	6	8	11	15	6	7	10	12	15
6.5-	4	6	8	11	14	6	7	10	13	17
7.5-	5	6	8	12	17	6	7	10	15	19
8.5-	5	6	9	14	19	6	7	11	17	24
9.5-	5	6	10	16	22	6	8	12	19	24
10.5-	6	7	10	17	25	7	8	12	20	29
11.5-	5	7	11	19	26	6	9	13	20	25
12.5-	5	6	10	18	25	7	9	14	23	30
13.5-	5	6	10	17	22	8	10	15	22	28
14.5-	4	6	9	19	26	8	11	16	24	30
15.5-	4	5	9	20	27	8	10	15	23	27
16.5-	4	5	8	14	20	9	12	16	26	31
17.5-24.4	4	5	10	18	25	9	12	17	25	31

[a]Based on data obtained using Lange skinfold calipers on white subjects included in the Ten State Nutrition Survey, 1968-1970.

children and this tendency to overfeed may be greater if both parents are obese. There is strong evidence that such environmental pressures do occur in these types of families. Hence, whether a strong family history implies a genetic etiology remains an open question. Regardless of the cause, however, a family history of obesity must immediately alert the physician to the fact that the patient is particularly at risk. Since there is little that can be done about the genetic problem, attempts to control the "energy environment," sometimes even prophylactically, should be made.

Once the diagnosis of obesity is made and its type suspected, the patient should be examined for organic diseases that are associated with obesity and, more important, for complications that are known to result from obesity itself. It is often said that a complete endocrine workup should be undertaken in very obese individuals. This is rarely necessary. If no other signs or symptoms of endocrine disease are present, it is unlikely that endocrine dysfunction is the cause of the obesity. Other rare causes of obesity, such as hypothalamic disease, should be readily apparent on careful history and physical examination. What is often not done for very obese patients, and what should be done, is a careful search for early evidence of complications. History of cardiovascular disease, serum lipid levels, blood pressure both at rest and during exercise, stress test, electrocardiogram, and glucose tolerance tests should all be examined. Even if all are negative, important baseline information will have been attained. If any is positive, specific therapy may be indicated and weight reduction becomes more urgent. To be sure, the slightly overweight individual can be put directly on a diet, but moderate or severe obesity should be handled as a serious medical problem meriting careful diagnosis, including a search for potential complications, and equally careful treatment.

CONTROL OF OBESITY

In order to control obesity and its subsequent complications both preventive and therapeutic methods must be employed.

Prevention

Prevention is the best and often the easiest way to control the problem of obesity. A routine physical examination should include weight for height and fatfold thickness measured serially. Any rate of increase above what would be expected should be considered a warning sign, even if the person is not yet obese. Moderate caloric restriction, increased exercise, and minor changes in lifestyle may be all that is necessary at this point. However, the physician should be alert to identify individuals at risk for obesity. Table 3 lists several signs that are helpful in determining the likelihood that obesity may develop.

The prevention of childhood and adolescent obesity may be the key to controlling the most malignant form of obesity—hyperplastic obesity. Since fat cell number is determined during these periods, any tendency to obesity at these times of life should be vigorously resisted. Parents should be alerted to the dangers to their children and a balanced diet, restricted in calories, which maintains growth but prevents obesity, should be prescribed. During adolescence the problem is more difficult because the eating patterns of adolescents are sometimes unconventional and often difficult to change. The physician should work *with* the adolescent to develop an acceptable

Table 3.   Risk factors for obesity

Family history of obesity
Obesity present in childhood
Change in lifestyle
  More sedentary occupation
  Increased consumption of alcohol
  Change in pattern of meal consumption
  Increase in snacking pattern
Major family or personal crisis

diet that fits within the adolescent lifestyle and controls calories sufficiently to control weight gain and still permit the adolescent growth spurt. Although this sounds complicated, it is really quite simple. It requires a moderate restriction of calories, to 70 to 80% of the recommended daily allowance for an adolescent of that sex and height, and meticulous attention to providing adequate amounts of such essential nutrients as iron. If caloric restriction cannot be achieved without compromising other nutrients, then supplements should be given during this period of life.

Obesity often begins to develop in early middle life; in men after they settle into a job (often in an office) and begin to raise a family, in women often after the birth of the first or second child. People who have a family history of obesity or who have been obese during childhood are especially at risk. Changes in lifestyle, such as the acquisition of a more sedentary job, an increase in the consumption of alcohol, eating more in restaurants —especially fast-food chains— and major family crises are also danger signs. These people should be warned that they are potentially obese and that it is extremely important that they not gain weight. They should be told that keeping weight down at this stage is much easier than taking it off later.

Unfortunately, these are the years when visits to a physician are fewest. Both obstetricians and pediatricians see families during this period. More people are going to family practitioners either for obstetrical or pediatric care or for the management of their own illnesses. Thus, certain physicians are finding themselves more and more in a position to take preventive measures against obesity, and should take advantage of the opportunity. Women should be encouraged to revert to their prepregnancy weight after childbirth. There is evidence that, besides its advantages to the infant, breast feeding can help a mother resume her prepregnancy weight more efficiently than bottle feeding. Thus, both for the sake of the mother and for the sake of the infant, breast feeding should be encouraged. If the mother has a tendency to obesity or is not losing weight after her delivery, mild caloric restriction that provides adequate amounts of essential nutrients will often be effective. If the problem of postpartum obesity in women and "middle-aged spread" in men can be prevented, many people might be spared a life of constant dieting.

Treatment of Obesity

The moderately obese patient has a potentially serious problem and should be treated accordingly. The person who is grossly obese is suffering from a disease that may lead to life-threatening complications. Both the physican and the patient must understand that losing weight and keeping it off is at best a difficult task; the patient must know what to expect and must understand that there will be periods of disappointment. But he must also be made to realize how important it is that the weight loss be maintained. The physician should help the patient set realistic goals. These goals depend in part on the nature and severity of the obesity and whether complications are present. Hence the goal will vary with the individual and the exact nature of the problem. The 350 lb person who has been obese from childhood is unlikely to be able to attain a weight of 150 to 175 lb and to maintain that weight for the rest of his life. Such a person is likely to have a hyperplastic adipose depot and therefore will never be able to achieve normal weight with adipocytes of normal size and number. This should be explained and more moderate goals should be set. It may be better for this person to get down to 250 lb and remain at that weight than to constantly "see-saw" between 175 and 350 lb.

After a careful history is recorded, a physical examination and appropriate laboratory tests must be performed with a view toward ruling out the complications of obesity. Table 4 lists the tests and examinations that should be made to determine whether known risk factors, such as hypertension, hyperlipidemia, and diabetes are present. Once this is done,

Table 4.   Determining complications of obesity

Blood pressure
Serum cholesterol and triglycerides
Glucose tolerance test
Electrocardiogram
Stress test

realistic goals can be set for the particular patient. If the tests indicate the presence of one or more complications, then the goal is weight reduction until the complication is adequately under control. For example, the 250 lb man with a blood pressure of 180/105, a serum cholesterol of 350, and an abnormal glucose tolerance test should lose weight until these abnormalities are markedly reduced or eradicated or until no further weight loss is attainable. A vigorous approach to weight reduction must be undertaken. By contrast,the same 250 lb man with a blood pressure of 120/80, a serum cholesterol of 185, and a normal glucose tolerance test can be approached more slowly and more moderate goals can be progressively set. From the standpoint of the patient's health, I cannot stress this point too strongly. It is the complications, and not obesity itself, which kill. Hence patients with these complications must be viewed differently from those without them.

Almost every mode of therapy employed in medical practice, and many not usually employed, have been tried in treating obesity. Controlling caloric intake and expenditure has always been and still remains the mainstay of therapy.

All of the various diet plans, when they work, owe their success to the establishment of an over-all negative caloric balance. The success of one over another depends entirely on the motivation of the patient to try and to maintain one type of regimen rather than another. Regardless of its claims, there is no evidence that any diet that works does so by any mechanism other than caloric reduction. However, since millions of people are constantly experimenting with one diet or another, the next section will be devoted to an evaluation of the various types of diets currently in use.

Recently, it has been recognized that since obesity often results from a change in lifestyle, redirecting the individual's lifestyle by behavior modification in such a way as to reduce caloric intake and increase energy expenditure often results in lasting weight reduction. Behavior modification, especially in a group setting, has been very effective. This approach, in an abridged fashion, is probably the major reason for the success of Weight Watchers. There are a number of competent psychiatrists and psychologists employing these techniques, and clinics are being established using the same principles. Fundamentally what is done is that patients are made aware of those habits peculiar to themselves which lead to overeating. Often patients do this by maintaining a diary, which is then examined in detail by themselves, their peers, and the therapist. A plan is evolved by which behavior patterns are changed gradually in a manner acceptable to the patient and consistent with the goal of reducing caloric intake. For example, if the person watches the Monday night football game and consumes 2 lb of peanuts and four bottles of beer, the substitution of a bowl of fruit and light beer or iced tea or coffee can save hundreds of calories. The patient may not have realized what he or she was doing and the change might be readily accepted. Several distinct changes such as this can result in reduction in caloric intake in excess of 1000 cal/day, and over time may establish a pattern of living that is compatible with a stable reduced weight.

Exercise has been receiving more and more attention as a method of weight reduction. While increasing exercise as a way of expending calories is an excellent adjunct to dietary management, it is in itself not a definitive treatment. Exercise is much more important in prevention and maintenance than in weight reduction. The type of exercise is very important. Dynamic exercises, such as swimming, cycling, walking, and jogging, are much better than static exercises, such as weight lifting, pushups, situps, etc. Table 5 gives the caloric expenditure of various forms of exercise.

Almost every type of drug has been tried in the treatment of obesity. Appetite depressants, metabolic stimulants, amphetamines, and hormones each has had its vogue. Some still have their advocates. None works in the long run; all have side effects, some serious. For this reason, they should not be used in the management of obesity.

Table 5. Calorie expenditures per hour for different activities[a]

Activity	Calories Expended per Hour of Continuous Exercise
Bicycle riding	200–600
Walking moderately fast	200–300
Football	560
Soccer	560
Frisbee	200
Basketball	500
Tennis	500–700
Volleyball	300
Swimming	300–600
Dancing	200–400
Jogging	400–500
Skiing	
Cross country	650–1000
Downhill	350–500

[a] Based on an individual weighing approximately 130–150 lb. More calories will be expended if heavier.

Surgical therapy has also been used. The current surgical procedure is intestinal bypass. This procedure produces severe side effects, such as intractable diarrhea with electrolyte problems and fatty liver which may progress to cirrhosis. Long-term follow-up experience has for the most part been poor. In my judgement, there is almost no indication for this operation. Other operations, such as wiring the mouth or teeth, have been used in the past; none has had any good long-term results.

It should be clear that there is no easy approach to the treatment of obesity. Dietary therapy is still the best approach. Unfortunately, there is no easy way to diet. The reason that fad diets come and go is that although they are easy for some patients to use in initial weight loss, they cannot be indefinitely maintained, and hence they ultimately fail. The best diet is one that will allow the person to eat as normally as possible and yet reduce his or her caloric intake. A number of these are available.

Dietary Management of Obesity

The cornerstone of any obesity regimen is the diet. Any successful diet must ultimately result in a reduced intake of calories. This reduction can be achieved either by limiting the quantity of food or by altering the quality of the over-all diet so that the individual foods are lower in calories. I believe deceiving the patient by prescribing a diet that purports to operate on any other principle is poor medical practice and rarely results in lasting benefit. When the physician deceives himself not only is it poor practice, but it demonstrates a gaping chasm in medical education. Since all three macronutrients, fat, carbohydrate, and protein, can be burned as energy or converted to adipose tissue, any calorie, regardless of its source, is potentially fat tissue. When caloric intake is reduced to a level below caloric expenditure, body fat begins to break down to make up the deficit. Fat is never burned exclusively; carbohydrate stores in the form of glycogen, and tissue protein (lean body mass) also are consumed. The premise under which many of the unusual diets operate is that one can increase the rate of adipose tissue breakdown while decreasing or sparing the loss of lean body mass. If this were true, certainly the diet that accomplished it would be useful. However, there is no evidence that there is any significant difference between high carbohydrate and low carbohydrate, high fat and low fat, high protein and low protein diets when compared on a calorie for calorie basis. And yet, each week a new diet becomes the rage. Atkins or Stillman, high carbohydrate or low carbohydrate, high protein, protein powder, or hydrolyzed protein, high alcohol, and most recently Scarsdale. Many of these diets will result in weight loss, sometimes even rapid weight loss. The reason, however, is that the intake of calories is reduced, some-

times because the diet itself limits calories (Scarsdale) and sometimes
because the very nature of the diet results in a reduction of food intake
(Atkins or "grapefruit"). Some of these diets can be dangerous, especially
if sustained for a long time. In addition, all of these diets suffer from
the same primary difficulty—the weight loss is usually rapidly regained
when the individual is finished dieting and returns to the previous eating
habits.

Unusual or "fad" diets can be separated into two major groups—those
that limit calories and those that allow unlimited calories. The first group
cuts out all foods that are high in calories but permits the person to eat
as much as he or she wants of whatever is left. If the permissible foods
supply adequate amounts of the essential nutrients, these diets are all
usable and, depending on palatability, variety, and personal preferences,
will have varied success. Many of these diets, however, are so constructed
that the "forbidden lists" prevent the person from consuming adequate
amounts of both macronutrients and micronutrients.

The currently popular Scarsdale diet is an example of the low calorie
approach. The menu is rigidly set forth. It is calculated to provide 1200-
1500 cal/day. Almost all carbohydrate and significant amounts of fat are
forbidden. Hence, it is a relatively high protein diet. The diet is such that
iron, unless consumed in fortified foods, is at best marginal. Calcium
requirements also are not adequately met on this diet. Hence the diet,
though effective and reasonably safe over a short period, must be abandoned
very soon. I will venture to predict that most patients who have lost weight
on this diet will return to previous eating patterns and eventually regain
most if not all of the weight. The diet will then simply fade out of popular-
ity as literally hundreds of similar diets have done. What is more disturbing,
perhaps, is that the same people who proclaimed this diet a success will be
trying the next one very soon and proclaiming it a success also.

A much more dangerous example of this type of unbalanced diet is
the use of liquid hydrolyzed protein as either the sole source or the major
source of calories. Over 50 deaths have been reported in connection with
this type of diet. These hydrolyzed proteins make no physiologic sense
since there is no evidence that protein digestion is in anyway impaired in
obese individuals. The protein source is often collagen, a protein with an
inadequate amount of certain essential amino acids. The only reason that
I can see for the use of such preparations is that they are cheap. A number
of patients who have died after using these preparations have had hypokalemia or other electrolyte abnormalities. Others have died with no apparent
explanation. Some have been "under a physicians care," the nature of
which I cannot imagine.

The protein powders added to a glass of skimmed milk as one meal, although they supply reduced calories in an unbalanced manner, are much less dangerous than the liquid hydrolyzed protein. They are usually made from casein, which is a complete protein, and in the way that they are used are probably safe for persons with no complicating disease. Patients with renal disease or reduced renal function should never be placed on a diet very high in protein. The kidney simply may not be able to handle the increased nitrogen load.

Finally, the complete or modified fast represents the calorie limited diet in its extreme form. As I pointed out in Chapter 5, the body makes a series of complex adaptive responses to fasting. Many of these can lead to undesirable symptoms and some of these symptoms may appear in obese individuals who are fasting. For this reason, a prolonged fasting regimen should be undertaken only in the hospital where the patient's cardiovascular and metabolic status can be monitored.

The second group of diets is represented by the Stillman diet, which consists almost solely of protein, or the Atkins diet, which consists of both protein and fat. Both restrict carbohydrates severely. Stillman tells you to "eat as much of the protein food as you want without stuffing yourself." Atkins presents his diet as a revolution and markets it as the "high calorie way to stay thin forever." Both of these diets are unbalanced and extremely high in protein, presenting a heavy nitrogen load to the kidney. In addition, the Atkins diet encourages the consumption of large amounts of saturated fat and cholesterol. As will be pointed out in the next chapter, a diet high in saturated fat should be avoided in general and should be avoided particularly by people with high blood lipid levels or with a history of cardiovascular disease. Moreover this high fat intake, combined with the reduced intake of carbohydrate, inevitably leads to ketosis. In fact, acetonuria is deemed essential by the proponents of the Atkins diet. Ketosis in itself can be troublesome in many people, producing headache, nausea, and vomiting. In certain people, ketosis may be extremely dangerous. For example, ketosis during early pregnancy may result in fetal damage.

Some people lose weight on these diets. Despite the fact that one is allowed to eat unlimited amounts of the permitted foods, many find they simply cannot tolerate large quantities of such foods. Hence, in reality, they are limiting their calories. In the long run, people find that they cannot maintain such an unbalanced diet for long and sooner or later they return to previous eating patterns and inevitably regain weight.

The dietary approach that is likely to produce the greatest long-term success is one which sets attainable goals, restricts calories, is nutritionally sound, and supplies the greatest variety of choices. Such a regimen requires

skill and patient guidance by the physician and cooperation and determination by the patient. The patient should be told the caloric content of
foods and how calories are converted to fat. It should be pointed out, for
example, that 1 lb of fat represents 3500 calories. Therefore, a reduction
of 500 cal/day should result in weight loss of approximately 1 lb/week.
Most adults will lose weight on a calorie intake ranging from 1000 to 1800
cal/day. This can be started immediately and will provide good nutrition
and adequate variety. A list of foods in various categories can be supplied
so that the patient can construct his or her daily menu by choosing a
prescribed number of foods from each category. An abbreviated example
is illustrated in Table 6. The patient can then pick a number of foods from
each category depending on the total number of calories being prescribed.
Table 7 demonstrates how this might be done for a patient consuming
1500 cal.

The following rules may help your patients avoid some of the common
problems of dieting:

1. Do not become discouraged when the more rapid initial weight loss
   begins to taper off as dieting proceeds.
2. Eat smaller portions five times a day instead of larger ones three times
   a day.
3. Use a smaller plate so that the smaller portions do not look too small.
4. Allow yourself a treat once a day.
5. Do not be fooled by high calorie "health food" snacks. Some of these
   snacks are just as high in calories as a chocolate bar.
6. Avoid luncheon meats or cold cuts, since these are usually very high in
   fat.

Table 6. Food categories for constructing a low calorie diet

1. Free foods	Lettuce, parsley, pickles, coffee, tea, bouillon
2. Vegetables	Almost all green and yellow vegetables
3. Fruits	Almost all fruits, dried fruits, berries, melons in prescribed amounts
4. Starch	Breads, rolls, crackers, starch, vegetables, cereals, alcohol
5. Meat	Beef, veal, lamb, pork, cheese, poultry, fish, seafood
6. Milk	Buttermilk, yogurt, skim milk
7. Fats	Creams, butter, certain meats, dressings

Table 7.   A balanced 1500 calorie diet

Basic Plan	Sample Menu	Free Foods
Morning		
List 3 = 1	½ small grapefruit	Coffee
List 5 = 1	1 medium egg	Artificial sweetener
List 4 = 2	1 slice whole wheat bread and 1½ cup puffed cereal	
List 7 = 1	1 tsp margarine	
List 6 = 1	1 cup (8 oz) skim milk	
Noon		
List 5 = 2	½ cup tuna (in water)	Lettuce
List 4 = 2	2 slices bread	Pickles
List 7 = 3	2 tsp. mayonnaise and 1 tsp oil	Lemon juice
List 2 = 1	3 slices tomato	Vinegar
List 3 = 1	½ cup diced pineapple	
Evening		
List 2 = 1	½ cup string beans	Lettuce
List 5 = 4	4 oz chicken (no skin)	Radishes
List 4 = 2	½ cup mashed potato and 4 oz fat free sherbert	Soy sauce
List 7 = 2	2 tsp margarine	Parsley
List 3 = 1	2 dates	
Snack		
List 6 = 1	8 oz skim milk	Coffee
List 4 = 1	1½ in. square sponge cake	

Keep in mind that dieting and weight maintenance are lifelong processes. Both the physician and the patient must accept this if maximum benefit is to be achieved.

Other factors, such as regular exercise, play a part in weight maintenance, but for the moderately and severely obese, long-term dietary regulation of some sort is mandatory.

RECOMMENDED READING

Asher, W. L., Ed., *Treating the Obese,* Medcom Press, New York, 1975.
Berland, T., *Rating the Diets,* Consumer Guide, Skokie, Ill., 1974.

Bjorntorp, P., A. Carlgren, B. Isaksson, M. Kootkiewski, B. Larsson, and L. Siöström, Effect of an Energy Reduced Dietary Regimen in Relation to Adipose Tissue Cellularity in Obese Women, *Am. J. Clin. Nutr.,* **28,** 445 (1975).

Brook, C. G. D., Evidence for a Sensitive Period in Adipose Cell Replication in Man, *Lancet,* **2,** 624 (1972).

Brook, C. G. D., J. K. Lloyd, and O. H. Wolff, Relation Between Age of Onset of Obesity and Size and Number of Adipose Cells, *Br. Med. J.,* **2,** 25 (1972).

Grinker, J., Behavioral and Metabolic Consequences of Weight Reduction, *J. Am. Dietet. Assoc.,* **62,** 30 (1973).

Jourdan, M., D. Goldbloom, S. Margen, and R. P. Bradfield, Differential Effects of Diet Composition and Weight Loss on Glucose Tolerance in Obese Women, *Am. J. Clin. Nutr.,* **27,** 1065, (1974).

Jourdan, M., S. Margen, and R. P. Bradfield, The Turnover Rate of Serum Glycerides in the Lipoproteins of Fasting Obese Women During Weight Loss, *Am. J. Clin. Nutr.,* **27,** 850 (1974).

Kalkhoff, R. K., H. J. Kim, J. Cerletty, and C. A. Ferrout, Metabolic Effects of Weight Loss in Obese Patients, *Diabetes,* **20,** 83 (1971).

Knittle, J. L., Obesity in Childhood: A Problem in Adipose Tissue Cellular Development, *J. Pediat.,* **81,** 1048 (1972).

Konshi, F., *Exercise Equivalents of Foods,* So. Illinois University Press, Carbondale, Ill., 1973.

Levitz, L. S., and A. J. Stunkard. A Therapeutic Coalition for Obesity: Behavior Modification and Patient Self Help, *Am. J. Psychiatry,* **131,** 423 (1974).

Salans, L. B., S. W. Cushman, and R. E. Weismann, Studies on Human Adipose Tissue: Adipose Cell Size and Number in Non-Obese and Obese Patients, *J. Clin Invest.,* **52,** 929 (1973).

Solow, C., P. M. Silberfarb, and L. Swift, Psychosocial Effects of Intestinal Bypass Surgery for Severe Obesity, *N. Engl. J. Med.,* **290,** 300 (1974).

Stuart, R. B., and P. Davis, *Slim Chance in a Fat World, Behavioral Control of Obesity,* Research Press, Champaign, Ill., 1972.

Weisman, R. E., Surgical Palliation of Massive Severe Obesity, *Am. J. Surg.,* **125,** 437 (1973).

Winick, M., *Childhood Obesity,* Wiley, New York, 1975.

13

EXCESS FAT

ARTERIOSCLEROSIS

Arteriosclerosis and its major pathological consequence, coronary artery disease, is a process that develops over a long period of time and is multifactorial in origin. The disease occurs as a consequence of the deposition of certain blood lipids (mainly cholesterol) into the lining of arteries. The deposited lipid first forms "streaks" within the intimal lining. These streaks gradually enlarge as more lipid is deposited, forming placques into which calcium may be deposited. The lumen of the vessel becomes more and more occluded and finally is blocked, causing necrosis of the tissue fed by the affected artery. In the case of the coronary artery, this results in a myocardial infarction.

There is evidence that this process begins relatively early in life and that the earliest lesions may already be present in males at the end of the second and the beginning of the third decade of life. Studies of battle casualties in the Viet Nam war revealed fatty streaks in a high proportion of young American servicemen. What is even more disturbing, however, is that these lesions were not noted at the same rate in casualties in previous wars. Hence indirect evidence suggests that arteriosclerosis is beginning earlier and earlier in life.

Many epidemiologic studies confirm the fact that the disease is multifactorial; that is, it is associated with a number of abnormalities which increase the risk of any given individual's being afflicted (Table 1).

The most important risk factors are cigarette smoking, hypertension, high serum lipids, particularly cholesterol, and diabetes. Obesity is also a risk factor, but its effect is indirect. Obesity increases the risk of hyper-

Table 1.   Risks for coronary artery disease

Cigarette smoking
Hypertension
Elevated serum lipids (cholesterol)
Diabetes

tension, elevated serum lipids, and diabetes, each of which, in turn, increases the risk of coronary artery disease.

Each of these risk factors is additive. Thus the heavy smoker with high blood pressure, high serum lipids, and diabetes is at maximal risk. As each of these factors is eliminated, the risk drops. Hence in an obese individual, it is possible to reduce three risk factors simultaneously by successful weight reduction. This is the major importance of obesity in coronary artery disease. Evidence from both epidemiologic and intervention studies overwhelmingly supports the thesis that the level of serum lipids, and especially of cholesterol, is at least in part under dietary control. For this reason, this chapter will focus on serum lipids and cholesterol as a risk factor for coronary artery disease. It should be understood, of course, that if any of the other risk factors is present it must be independently dealt with.

CONTROL OF SERUM LIPID LEVELS

Cholesterol is carried in the serum combined with other lipids and protein in a complex molecule called lipoprotein. The serum contains a number of the lipoproteins, and they are classified according to their density—high density lipoprotein (HDL), low density lipoprotein (LDL), and very low density lipoprotein (VLDL). Most of the cholesterol is in the form of LDL-cholesterol. This is what the usual serum cholesterol determination measures. High levels of cholesterol in this form are associated with an increased incidence of coronary artery disease.

The higher the cholesterol level, the greater the risk. There is no really normal value, only average values for a person in our population. In view of the fact that our population is one in which the incidence of coronary artery disease is alarmingly high, the so-called normal value (around 200 for a middle-aged male) is no doubt too high. Other things being equal, a person with a serum cholesterol of 150 is at lower risk than a person with a serum cholesterol level of 200 even though both have "normal" values.

Cholesterol is manufactured in the body and is also available in the diet.

The level in the blood is determined by availability from these two sources and is regulated by a kind of feedback mechanism. Thus, increased exogenous cholesterol will reduce endogenous synthesis. This feedback system, however, can be overwhelmed by ingestion of large amounts of saturated fat and cholesterol. Hence, at high baseline levels of ingestion, any increased intake will increase serum levels. The saturated fats in general will increase the serum cholesterol level whereas polyunsaturated fats will decrease the level. The prudent diet, which we shall discuss in detail, is a diet low in saturated fat and cholesterol and relatively high in polyunsaturated fat.

Recently, there have been a number of studies indicating that high density lipoprotein (HDL) is important in the removal and transport of cholesterol from tissue (and perhaps from the arterial wall itself) to the liver for subsequent transformation and excretion. Plasma HDL-cholesterol was *decreased* in conditions that have been associated with an increased risk of coronary artery disease (Figure 1). In a study done in 6859 people in five different population groups across the United States, the average HDL-cholesterol levels in persons known to have coronary artery disease were consistently lower than for persons without coronary heart disease.

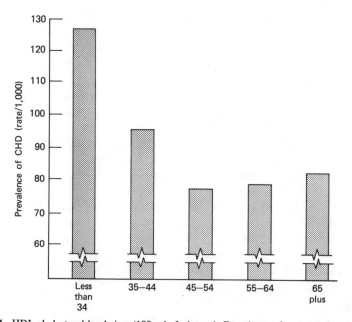

Figure 1. HDL cholesterol levels (mg/100 ml of plasma). Prevalence of coronary heart disease (CHD) according to plasma HDL cholesterol levels in men aged 50-69. The lower the HDL cholesterol level, the higher the risk of coronary heart disease. (Adapted from Castelli et al., *Circulation,* 55, 767 (1977).)

In several studies, runners and skiers have been found to have higher levels of HDL than similar individuals who do not participate in these activities. Hence one of the benefits of exercise appears to be that it increases the levels of this "protective" lipoprotein. If, as present evidence indicates, high levels of HDL-cholesterol are indeed protective against coronary artery disease, then it is extremely important for us to identify those factors which can increase the levels of HDL-cholesterol in plasma. The limited information available suggests that physical activity and weight loss are two such factors.

There is very little disagreement that high levels of LDL-cholesterol, especially when coupled with low levels of HDL-cholesterol, increase the risk of coronary artery disease. There is also general agreement that, since plasma cholesterol levels represent a balance between the amount manufactured by the body and the amount consumed in the diet, reducing the dietary intake of cholesterol and saturated fat will only partially lower plasma cholesterol. The reason for this is that endogenous production will increase. The amount of increased production, however, will vary from individual to individual and a new "steady state" will be achieved at lower plasma levels. What is not agreed upon is how much blood cholesterol can be lowered by consuming a diet low in cholesterol and saturated fat. A good rule of thumb is 15 to 20%, but this will vary from person to person and is especially dependent on the initial level. People with very high levels to start with will usually show greater drops with dietary control.

Recently, there has been a great deal of talk and very few data suggesting that other dietary factors may be involved in elevating serum cholesterol levels and hence in increasing the incidence of coronary artery disease. First on this list has been sugar. A few reports have suggested that sucrose per se can elevate serum cholesterol levels. A larger number of studies have shown no effect. At best, one can say that a small percentage of the population may react in this way. Thus, restricting sugar in all patients with hypercholesterolemia is not warranted. A short therapeutic trial of sugar restriction can be tried to determine if sucrose limitation will have any benefit. The major danger of large amounts of sugar in the diet is that it supplies a sweet tasting, low bulk source of calories and may in that way contribute to obesity.

A second class of substances that have been suggested to influence serum cholesterol levels is fiber. It has been suggested that both bran (the outer layer of cereal grains) and pectin (found in fruits and vegetables) have a lowering effect on serum cholesterol levels. Available evidence is too limited to draw any definite conclusions, but the thesis is being currently tested in several centers both here and abroad.

There is some evidence that consuming *small amounts* of alcohol daily may offer some protection against coronary artery disease and that this protection is mediated by affecting serum lipid levels. The data suggest that rather than lowering LDL-cholesterol, moderate alcohol consumption elevated HDL-cholesterol levels. While this is not yet proven, it is tempting to speculate that the preventive role of light alcohol consumption may be mediated by means of increases in HDL.

A final nutrient about which there has been much discussion is vitamin E. Because of its antioxidant properties, it has been suggested that vitamin E may protect the heart tissue from damage in coronary insufficiency. Although there might be some theoretical reasons why this could be true, there are no well controlled clinical studies which demonstrate that this actually happens. Although there is probably no danger in using moderate doses of vitamin E in patients with high risk for coronary heart disease (CHD), it is no substitute for direct interventions aimed at reducing each individual risk factor.

Thus for the physician two problems must be dealt with if the high incidence of CHD is to be reduced. Patients who *potentially* may become high risk individuals must be identified and prevented from developing the known risk factors. Patients who already have one or more risk factors must be helped to reduce that risk. In dealing with the first problem, it is important to consider a number of factors (Table 2).

The person with a poor family history for any of the risk factors must be considered a potential candidate for developing these risk factors himself. Preventive dietary therapy and careful follow-up are indicated. For the second type of individual, the one who already is at risk, intervention is mandatory. Cigarette smoking should be vigorously opposed; hypertension should be effectively managed; weight loss should be encouraged through diet and exercise; diabetes should be controlled, and a prudent diet low in cholesterol and saturated fat should be encouraged.

THE PRUDENT DIET

The so-called prudent diet, which is essentially a diet low in saturated fat and cholesterol and relatively high in polyunsaturated fat, was originally devised by Norman Jolliffe when he was directing the "anticoronary club"

Table 2.   Individuals with "risk potential"

Family history of CHD
Family history of hyperlipidemia
Family history of diabetes
Overweight
Family history of hypertension

in the Bureau of Nutrition of the New York City Health Department. Subsequently, with some modifications, it has been adopted by the American Heart Association and at present is widely employed for the prevention of coronary artery disease particularly in patients with high levels of serum cholesterol.

The diet attempts to modify a single nutrient—fat. It limits the *amount* and the *kind* of fat consumed. In this diet fat contributes less than one-third of the total calories, and at least twice as much polyunsaturated fat as saturated fat (a P:S ratio greater than 2) is recommended. In addition, cholesterol intake is kept under 300 mg/day. To achieve this, certain dietary guidelines must be followed. In general, foods from vegetable sources are more acceptable in the prudent diet than those from animal sources because both saturated fat and cholesterol are more common in foods from animal sources. The greatest concentration of cholesterol is found in eggs and organ meats (fowl eggs, fish roe, beef, calf, or chicken livers, kidneys, heart, and brains). Table 3 lists the approximate cholesterol content of common meats. It is important to note that the more fat on the meat, the greater the amount of cholesterol. Because certain meats can never be lean and trimmed enough, they are not recommended for regular use in the prudent diet. Table 4 lists those high fat meats as well as the lean cuts which are recommended. Fruits, vegetables, grains and grain products (such as breads, pastas, breakfast cereals, rice, etc.), and beans are virtually fat free. In some cases, however, fat is added during

Table 3. Average cholesterol content of common meats

Food	Cholesterol (mg)
1. Liver (3 oz)	372
2. Egg (large)	252
3. Shrimp, canned (3 oz)	128
4. Veal (3 oz)	86
5. Lamb (3 oz)	83
6. Beef (3 oz)	80
7. Pork (3 oz)	76
8. Lobster (3 oz)	72
9. Chicken ($1/2$ breast, no skin)	63
10. Clams, canned ($1/2$ cup)	50
11. Chicken (1 drumstick)	39
12. Fish, fillet (3 oz)	34–75

Table 4. Distribution of fats in common foods

High in Polyunsaturated Fats	Moderately High in Polyunsaturated Fats	High in Monounsaturated Fats	High in Saturated Fats	High in Cholesterol
Safflower oil	Soybean oil	Peanut oil	Meats high in fat: sausages, cold cuts, prime cuts, etc.	Egg yolks
Corn oil	Cottonseed oil	Peanuts and peanut butter		Liver
Soft margarine: made of corn oil	Other soft margarines	Olive oil	Chicken fat	Kidney
Walnuts	Commercial salad dressings	Olives	Meat drippings	Sweetbreads
Soybeans	Mayonnaise	Almonds	Lard	Brains
Sunflower seeds		Pecans	Hydrogenated shortening	Heart
Sesame seeds		Cashews	Stick margarines	Paté
Oils made from these seeds		Brazil nuts	Coconut oil	Caviar
		Avocados	Butter and products with dairy fat, e.g., cheese, cream, whole milk, ice cream, chocolate, bakery items	Dairy fats
				Products made with the above, e.g., cakes, pies, pastries, gravies, etc.

processing. If this is the case, the amount and kind should be determined and considered in the over-all diet plan. Certain plants, mainly seeds and nuts but also corn and other plants, contain fat. The most familiar products in this group are the vegetable oils and the margarines that are made from them. Here the kinds of fat become very important. The relatively unsaturated fats are more desirable. All natural fats are a mixture of saturated, monounsaturated, and polyunsaturated fat. The higher the ratio of polyunsaturated to saturated (P:S ratio) the better. Corn oil, for example, has a P:S ratio of 4. In general, the harder the fat the lower the P:S ratio. Thus, soft margarines have a higher P:S ratio than stick margarines. It should be noted that the fats in meats, poultry, and dairy products, while predominantly saturated, contain small amounts of polyunsaturated fat (see Table 4). The amount varies with each animal. For example, beef fat has an average P:S ratio of 1:18, pork 1:4 and chicken and fish 1:1. Thus, even gram for gram, certain animal fats are more acceptable than others.

Using the above general principles, the physician can now construct a general diet plan for a patient with high levels of serum lipids or with a family history of early coronary artery disease.

To limit the *amount* of cholesterol and saturated fat, consumption of certain animal products must be curtailed. The maximum amount of meat, poultry, or fish per day is 6 oz if total caloric intake is under 1500 cal, and 8 oz if caloric intake is greater. This level ensures a cholesterol intake of less than 300 mg/day and limits the amount of fat consumed primarily in saturated form. The red meats (beef, lamb, and pork) should be limited to 16 oz/week.

To this diet, 3 or 4 tablespoons (depending on whether 6 or 8 oz of meat are being consumed) of a high polyunsaturated fat should be consumed each day. This will ensure a dietary P:S ratio of 2:1 or higher. Egg yolks should be limited to two per week, whether eaten plain or in prepared foods. Egg whites and other foods that contain no fat can be consumed without any restriction as long as the total number of calories recommended is not exceeded.

The prudent diet is not very different from the way many people in many countries ordinarily eat. Moreover, the incidence of coronary artery disease in countries consuming this type of diet is much lower than the incidence in the United States.

CARCINOMA OF THE COLON AND BREAST

There is a certain amount of evidence, mostly epidemiologic, that at least two types of cancer, colon and breast, are associated with consumption of excessive amounts of fat in the diet.

There is a high incidence of these cancers in western industrialized countries, with the exception of Japan. In racial groups where the incidence of these types of cancer is low, moving to a western environment rapidly increases the incidence. Correlations with dietary constituents suggest that total dietary fat and total meat, especially beef, consumption correlate extremely well with the incidence of these cancers.

It is interesting that the incidence of cancer of the colon and breast correlates inversely with the incidence of cancer of the stomach, suggesting that certain factors promoting one type of cancer may protect against the other. For example, in Japan the over-all incidence of stomach cancer is high, whereas that of breast and colon cancer is low. However, among patients with colon cancer there is a very high incidence of consumption of western diets. By contrast, in individuals consuming such western diets, the incidence of stomach cancer is low.

A current hypothesis about the etiology of colon cancer claims that the high fat in the diet increases the concentration of bile acids and neutral steroids in the large bowel and also increases the concentration of certain colonic bacteria which metabolize these bile acids and neutral sterols to carcinogens or cocarcinogens or both. Although no carcinogen has yet been identified in colon carcinoma, active research in this area continues. Animal studies have shown that several bile acids are able to induce tumors at remote sites and that increasing the amount of bile salts experimentally in rats resulted in an increased incidence of colonic tumors. Other studies have shown that deoxycholic acid, lithocholic acid, cholic acid, and chenodeoxycholic acid also produce this result in germ-free and conventional rats.

The possible role of dietary fat in inducing cancer of the colon also has received some support from animal studies. Rats fed diets containing 20% lard or 20% corn oil had a higher incidence of DMH-induced colon tumors than rats fed diets with 5% lard or 5% corn oil. Similar results have been obtained by feeding rats a high beef, high fat diet or a high soybean protein, high corn oil diet.

Data among patients with cancer of the colon indicate that their stool contains increased amounts of bile acids and cholesterol metabolites and that their stool β-glucuronidase activity is elevated. Since many compounds, including potential carcinogens, are conjugated with glucuronide, the data imply that individuals with colonic cancer have a bacterial flora more active in such conjugation. Most of the experimental work relating diet to hormone-dependent cancers has been concerned with mammary cancer. Studies with animals have shown that restricting caloric intake inhibits development of mammary tumors, and that increasing the level of fat in the diet stimulates mammary tumor development. The effect of caloric restriction is a general one, influencing most kinds of tumors, whereas the stimulation by dietary fat is more selective for certain types of tumors.

The effect of dietary fat appears to be largely independent of caloric intake and the high fat diet is effective when given only after animals have been exposed to a carcinogen. This suggests that dietary fat acts as a promoting agent, producing a more favorable environment for the development of latent tumor cells. Unsaturated fats seem to be more effective than saturated fats in promoting mammary tumorigenesis, but it is not certain whether this difference is related to their content of essential fatty acids.

Epidemiological data on human populations show a strong positive correlation between dietary fat intake and age-adjusted mortality from breast cancer in different countries of the world. Similar, but somewhat weaker, correlations have been observed between fat intake and certain other types of cancer, including prostatic cancer and ovarian cancer. Breast cancer mortality is also positively correlated with total caloric intake, and with intakes of animal protein and simple sugars. These epidemiological data provide clues to the possible influence of different dietary components on carcinogenesis, which are being explored with the use of animal models.

Thus, while the evidence is by no means complete, there is sufficient reason to believe that high levels of dietary fat, in this case total fat, may in some way contribute to developing cancer of the colon and perhaps cancer of the breast as well. It would be hard to make any kind of dietary recommendations based on these data alone. However, since it seems clear that Americans consume too much fat in their diets, these data provide an added impetus for reducing the over-all fat consumption by our population.

RECOMMENDED READING

Bortz, W. M., The Pathogenesis of Hypercholesterolemia, *Ann. Int. Med.,* **80**, 738 (1974).

Christakis, G., Designing a New American Nutritional Pattern, *Food Tech.,* **28**, 17 (1974).

Connor, W. E., and S. L. Connor, Nutrition Management of Hyperlipidemias, in M. Winick, Ed., *Nutritional Management of Genetic Disorders,* Wiley, New York, 1979.

Frederickson, D. S., in *Harrison's Principles of Medicine,* T. Wintrobe, Ed., McGraw-Hill, New York, 1974.

Grundy, S. M., Effect of Polyunsaturated Fats on Lipid Metabolism in Patients with Hypertriglyceridemia, *J. Clin. Invest.,* **55**, 269 (1975).

Jenkins, D. A., A. R. Leeds, C. Newton, and J. H. Cummings, Effect of Pectin, Guar Gum, and Wheat Fiber on Serum-Cholesterol, *Lancet,* **1**, 1116 (1975).

Lauer, R. M., W. Connor, P. Leaverton, M. A. Reiter, and W. R. Clarke, Coronary Heart Disease Risk Factors in School Children: The Muscatine Study, *J. Pediat.,* **86**, 697 (1975).

Livingston, G. E., The Prudent Diet: What? Why? How?, *Food Tech.,* **28**, 16 (1974).

Reiser, R., Saturated Fat in the Diet and Serum Cholesterol Concentration. A Critical Examination of the Literature, *Am. J. Clin. Nutr.,* **26**, 524 (1973).

Wilmore, J. H., and J. J. McNamara, Prevalence of Coronary Heart Disease Risk Factors in Boys 8 to 12 Years of Age, *J. Pediat.,* **84**, 527 (1974).

14

EXCESS CARBOHYDRATE

The American diet in general is not relatively high in carbohydrate. On the contrary, most nutritionists believe that the carbohydrate content of our diet should increase or remain the same whereas the fat content and protein content should be reduced. Hence in this chapter we are concerned not with excess total carbohydrate but rather with excess of certain forms of carbohydrate, particularly refined sugar or sucrose, which is consumed by itself and added to many foods.

SUCROSE

Sucrose is used widely in the food industry—in baking, confection making, and soft drink preparation. Consumption has increased considerably since the beginning of the century and many people have been greatly concerned that our high sucrose consumption may be detrimental to our health, especially in the areas of dental caries, obesity, diabetes, atherosclerosis, and hypoglycemia. As we shall see, some of these concerns are much more valid than others.

Dental Caries

Dental caries is an infectious disease caused by particular metabolic products of bacteria that act at the tooth surface. The sequence of events involves:

1. An oral bacterial flora that contains bacteria of a particular type—mainly streptococcus mutans.

2. A substrate that the bacteria can metabolize to form a variety of acids and to use in construction of a complex polysaccharide "shield" known as plaque, which adheres to the tooth surface.

3. A tooth surface that is relatively dissolvable by the acids produced.

Figure 1 is a diagrammatic representation of how dental caries are produced.

Hence dental caries is a complex multifactorial disease involving bacteria, sugar, and the fundamental erosion resistance of the tooth enamel. The amount of sucrose consumed is one element in the formation of dental caries. However it is not just the total quantity of sucrose but the form in which the sucrose is presented to the teeth that is important. Sucrose is most dangerous from the standpoint of dental caries when consumed between meals, when in a sticky vehicle such as a candy or gum, when in acid media (soft drinks), and when administered in a constant drip (propping a bottle of sugar water in a baby's mouth).

Several methods have been recommended for preventing dental caries, each dealing with one of the three major aspects of the disease—substrate, bacteria, and basic tooth resistance. In the case of substrate, since sucrose is the worst offender attempts are being made to discourage sucrose intake, especially in its most cariogenic form. Sweetening agents other than sucrose are being employed. These consist of two types, natural agents, such as fructose and xylose (two other sugars) and aspartane (a peptide), and artificial agents, such as saccharin. There is some evidence that another natural agent, xylitol, a complex sugar, when used in chewing gum, may actually be anticariogenic. Finally, the practice of "bottle propping" should be discouraged, since this may lead to severe tooth decay and rampant dental caries (Figure 2).

From the standpoint of bacteria, meticulous dental hygiene, including frequent brushing and mouth washes, is extremely useful. Still in the research stage is the development of a vaccine against streptococcus mutans.

Perhaps the most successful public health approach to the control of dental caries is the attempt to increase the resistance of the tooth itself.

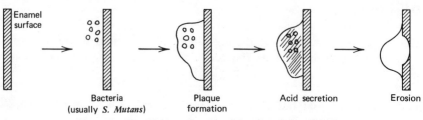

Figure 1. Simplified mechanism of dental caries production.

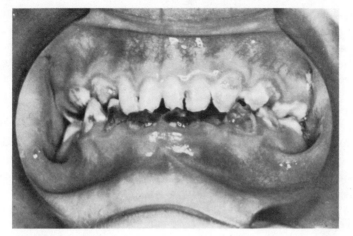

Figure 2. Nursing bottle syndrome; rampant destruction of deciduous teeth caused by bottle propping. (From Fomon, 1974.)

The major success in this approach has been the use of fluoride. The ingestion of 1 part per million (ppm) in drinking water and other fluids, or 0.5 mg/day for children, has been shown to reduce the incidence of dental caries markedly. In areas where water is either naturally or artificially fluoridated there has been a 50 to 70% reduction in dental caries. It should be noted that boiling water in aluminum pots reduces the fluoride content whereas boiling in teflon pots increases fluoride content.

There is little evidence that fluoride will protect the fetus from developing dental caries later. Fluoride is therefore not recommended during pregnancy, and recently it has been banned by the Food and Drug Administration from use in pregnant women. For the young infant, even before the teeth erupt, fluoride is extremely protective. Since fluoridation of water supplies varies throughout the United States and since most infant formulas add water at the plant or in the mother's home, the amount of fluoride in infant formula is erratic and unknown. Hence at present 0.25 to 0.5 mg/day of fluoride is recommended for young infants.

Fluoride acts by reducing the solubility of enamel after displacing hydroxide ions in the structure of hydroxy apatite. Although the major concentration of fluoride is in the surface enamel of the tooth, some fluoride also gets into the plaque and inhibits bacterial acid production.

When consumed in excessive amounts fluoride itself may be toxic; at 2 ppm over a prolonged period mottling of the tooth enamel may occur. While this mottling is cosmetically unpleasant it will have little effect on the tooth itself. Very high amounts (20 to 80 mg/day) can cause skeletal deformities.

Hence dental caries is a disease produced in part by overuse of sugar, mainly sucrose, particularly in an improper vehicle. In this sense, control of the amount and the type of sucrose ingested is very important. However, the two other aspects of prevention, proper oral hygiene and ingestion of fluoride, are equally important and should also be encouraged.

Obesity

It has been claimed that ingestion of large amounts of refined sugar per se can lead to obesity. While this is not true, since the induction of obesity is dependent on total calories and not on the source of those calories, sugar is a pleasant tasting, low bulk source of calories. Thus it is easy to consume a large number of "extra" calories by ingesting sugar. For example, a person who consumes six cups of coffee per day can increase caloric intake by several hundred calories simply by using sugar as a sweetener. Since sugar is added to most foods as a flavoring, not as a nutrient, we pay a caloric price for sweetness. Unless we recognize this and either reduce the intake of other calories or reduce our sugar intake we may consume too many total calories and thereby initiate obesity.

A second claim which is often made is that sugar, particularly sucrose, can induce a "sweet tooth" in a person, thereby making that person "crave" sweet tasting food. This, in turn, leads to an increased consumption of calories and subsequent obesity. The few studies that have been carried out do not bear this out. Obese adults do not show any preference for sweet tasting foods. On the contrary, they prefer less sweet solutions than lean individuals. Even after weight reduction they continue to prefer less sweet solutions. Obese children show the same pattern as obese adults but after weight reduction they show the same preferences as normal children. Young infants prefer sweet solutions shortly after birth and this preference seems to persist. Hence the evidence suggests that preference for sweet taste is innately present and that obese individuals seem to show less of this preference than lean individuals.

Diabetes

Because diabetes is a disease involving abnormalities in carbohydrate metabolism and because its treatment involves restriction of sugar, it has been claimed that high consumption of sugar over long periods can actually cause diabetes. There is no evidence at present to substantiate this claim. The only way in which this association may be valid is indirectly, as a result of obesity. As was just mentioned, sugar as a pleasant, low bulk source of calories may contribute to obesity. Obesity, in turn, is an extremely important risk factor in developing diabetes. However, as long as total caloric intake remains at or below recommended levels, sugar per se is not important in the etiology of diabetes.

Atherosclerosis

A few studies indicate that in certain individuals consumption of a sugar load will result in elevation in serum cholesterol levels. When the total number of studies is evaluated, it appears that this effect occurs in a relatively small number of individuals. Hence reducing the over-all sugar content of our diet cannot be expected to result in any significant reduction in the over-all incidence of coronary artery disease. However, in any given patient with high levels of serum cholesterol, a trial of sugar restriction may be undertaken for a short period to see if there is any effect. If this is done, it should come after the patient has been on a prudent diet and gotten the maximum cholesterol lowering effect from restricting animal fat. A 1 to 2 week trial of sucrose restriction should tell the physician whether further lowering of serum cholesterol will occur and if so how much. At that point a decision can be made whether to reinstitute sugar in the diet.

Hypoglycemia

The term hypoglycemia has recently been used by both physicians and the general public to explain a variety of nonspecific symptoms. Hypoglycemia, of course, is not a diagnosis but a biochemical response by which a variety of diseases may manifest themselves. Blood glucose levels are usually maintained within narrow limits. After eating, the rise in blood glucose is blunted by the secretion of insulin. Conversely, starvation produces a release of liver glycogen and the production of glucose from gluconeogenesis. When blood glucose falls below certain critical levels, insulin secretion is impeded and catecholamines, glucagon, glucocorticoids, and growth hormone are secreted. It is the release of catecholamines that causes the early symptoms of hypoglycemia. These include sweating, palpitation, anxiety, and weakness. The symptoms themselves are not specific for hypoglycemia and may occur under a variety of conditions which elevate catecholamine release.

This symptom complex usually occurs only at blood glucose levels of 40 mg/dl or below. As the blood glucose level continues to fall, signs of central nervous system impairment may appear—confusion, blurred vision, amnesia, bizarre behavior, and depressed intellectual function. If hypoglycemia becomes too severe, hypothermia, convulsions, and coma may result.

It is the early, nonspecific symptoms associated with the release of catecholamines that are often diagnosed as hypoglycemia. The diagnosis is made much too frequently. In order to make this diagnosis, one must demonstrate a blood sugar level below 40 mg/dl *at the time* symptoms occur *and* one must demonstrate the alleviation of symptoms with the restoration of normal blood glucose levels.

Hypoglycemic disorders can be divided into two broad categories (Table 1), reactive (food stimulated), occurring 2 to 4 hours after meals, and fasting (food deprived), occurring unassociated with meals. By far the most common cause of hypoglycemia is the use of hypoglycemic drugs (insulin, sulfonylureas) for the treatment of diabetes. All of the other causes in both groups are extremely rare.

Reactive Hypoglycemias

The reactive or food stimulated hypoglycemias have gained a great deal of notoriety in the lay press and are often misdiagnosed by physicians. To establish the diagnosis a 5 hour glucose tolerance test should be undertaken. However, a number of factors must be taken into account when carrying out this test. These include age of the patient, presence of obesity, use of medications, diet, presence of concurrent illness, physical inactivity, and hypokalemia. If these factors are not considered, the diagnosis of hypoglycemia may be made fallaciously. Blood glucose levels may fall to 40 mg/dl in normal individuals during a 5 hour glucose tolerance test and hence such levels are not diagnostic unless symptoms occur at the time that these low levels are manifest. If the patient demonstrates reactive

Table 1.   Classification of hypoglycemias

Reactive (food stimulated)	Alimentary
	Early diabetes
Fasting (food deprived)	Drugs
	Alcohol
	Hormone deficiency
	Liver disease
	Congenital enzyme deficiency
	Insulinoma
	Neonatal hypoglycemia

hypoglycemia it is usually possible to diagnose the cause by carefully noting the time after ingestion of the oral load when the blood sugar reaches its lowest level. In early diabetes blood glucose reaches its lowest level at about 4 hours. By contrast, in alimentary reactive hypoglycemia and in the so-called "idiopathic" reactive hypoglycemia this occurs at about 2 hours after loading.

Once the diagnosis of alimentary hypoglycemia is made, such organic disease as postgastrectomy syndrome or vagotomy must be ruled out. Only after they have been ruled out should the diagnosis of "idiopathic hypoglycemia" be made.

The hypoglycemia of early diabetes may be treated with a diabetic diet, weight reduction, or both. By contrast, alimentary hypoglycemia is usually controlled by the ingestion of multiple small meals.

Fasting Hypoglycemias

The fasting hypoglycemias frequently are characterized by signs of central nervous system dysfunction without noticeable symptoms of catecolamine excess.

Drugs. Insulin or sulfonylureas administered either by the patient or by the physician are the most common cause of hypoglycemia, and in any diabetic receiving such therapy the diagnosis of hypoglycemia must be considered when signs of central nervous system depression or of excess catecholamine secretion are present.

Alcohol. Profound hypoglycemia may occur after alcohol ingestion both in the chronic malnourished alcoholic and in the weekend "binge" drinker. Occasionally it is also seen in the healthy child after accidental ingestion of alcohol. Since the susceptibility to alcohol-induced hypoglycemia increases as liver glycogen stores decrease, the risk is greatest when the patient has undergone a period of fasting before alcohol ingestion.

Deficiency of hyperglycemic hormones. This diagnosis should be readily apparent from the symptoms of the basic hormone defect (growth hormone or glucocorticoid or both) and can be confirmed by employing the appropriate stimulation tests.

Liver disease. Severe liver disease, such as fulminant hepatic necrosis, advanced cirrhosis, or malignancy, may result in moderate hypoglycemia due to impairment of gluconeogenesis and glycogenesis.

Congenital enzyme deficiencies. On very rare occasions deficiency of certain hepatic enzymes involved in glycogenolysis or gluconeogensis may result in hypoglycemia. However, the constellation of biochemical abnormalities induced by these diseases will usually suggest the diagnosis.

Nonpancreatic tumors. Sometimes a very large tumor (over 1 kg) located in the abdomen or chest will induce symptoms of hypoglycemia. These

---

are readily diagnosed on physical examination or X-ray and the hypoglycemic symptoms disappear when the tumor is removed.

Insulinoma. Insulin-secreting tumors of the pancreas are most common in patients over 50 years of age. Symptoms of hypoglycemia are intermittent, are usually progressive, and often begin 2 years or more before the diagnosis is made. Impairment of central nervous system function is often the presenting complaint, while the nonspecific symptoms of excess catecholamines go unrecognized. The diagnosis depends on the repeated demonstration of low blood glucose levels (40 mg/dl or less) and an elevated plasma insulin level at the time of spontaneous symptoms. This is sometimes demonstrable by fasting the patient for 72 hours *in the hospital.* Once the diagnosis of insulinoma has been confirmed and it has been angiographically localized, surgical removal should be undertaken.

Infants and Children

Certain hypoglycemic disorders are confined to the neonate or young infant. Transient neonatal hypoglycemia (blood glucose under 20 mg/dl) may appear as early as hours after birth in infants of diabetic mothers or in infants with erythroblastosis fetalis. Infants who are very small as a result of prematurity or intrauterine growth failure, and some very large infants, may exhibit hypoglycemia during the first few days of life. Such hypoglycemia can be controlled with a few days of supportive therapy.

Some children, usually between 18 months and 5 years of age, show episodes of hypoglycemia with concurrent ketosis. The disease is usually self limiting and can be controlled with frequent feedings until the hypoglycemia spontaneously remits.

In summary, hypoglycemia, especially reactive hypoglycemia, is a diagnosis that is made too often. In order for a valid diagnosis to be made, blood glucose levels should drop below 40 mg/dl 2 hours after a glucose load or test meal and symptoms should appear at that time. If these criteria are used, the disease is quite rare. Symptoms that occur during food deprivations are potentially more serious, may have a variety of causes, and usually require special diagnostic tests.

LACTOSE

Lactose, or milk sugar, is the major carbohydrate in the milk of all mammals except the California sea lion. During the digestive process it is cleaved by the enzyme lactase to glucose and galactose, which are then absorbed into the body. If this cleavage does not take place, lactose is carried intact into the lower bowel. Hence glucose is not absorbed and the blood glucose does not change. Moreover the lactose in the large bowel is osmotically active, drawing in water, and is fermented by bacteria to produce acids and gases. A number of terms have been employed to describe this syndrome so I shall define the terms most commonly used.

Lactose intolerance refers to the occurrence of gastrointestinal symptoms, such as flatulence, bloating, abdominal cramps, or watery diarrhea, after the ingestion of a test dose of lactose (50 g or 2 g/kg in aqueous solution). *Lactose malabsorption* refers to the failure to achieve a blood glucose increase of 20 mg/dl or more at some point between 15 and 60 minutes after a test dose of lactose. *Lactase deficiency* refers to abnormally low lactase activity in duodenal or jejunal mucosa obtained by peroral biopsy. Congenital lactase deficiency is rare; lactase deficiency is much more commonly encountered in children when there is an anatomic lesion of the intestinal mucosa caused by celiac disease, a viral, bacterial, or parasitic infection, or protein-calorie malnutrition. In humans of most races throughout the world (Scandinavians and West Europeans are the exception) lactase activity declines during childhood and a high proportion of healthy adults belonging to these races are lactase deficient. Lactose malabsorption is usually, but not always, indicative of lactase deficiency and the lactose tolerance test has been extensively used to investigate populations for the prevalence of lactase deficiency. Many, but not all, people with lactose malabsorption and lactase deficiency also have lactose intolerance. Lactose intolerance or malabsorption due to the primary adult form of lactase deficiency begins to appear after the age of about 5 years in children of African, Asian, and Latin American origin, and a year or so earlier in children from India and Thailand. There is some evidence to suggest that a decline in intestinal lactase activity may be delayed in children who continue to ingest large quantities of milk after weaning, but more research is needed to establish this. There has been controversy about the relation of lactose malabsorption and intolerance to milk intolerance. To consume the same amount of lactose used for the test dose (50 g) it would be necessary for a person to drink just over a liter of milk at one sitting—an amount that only the most avid milk drinkers are capable of drinking. There is some question whether individuals intolerant to such an unphysiological dose of lactose also have symptoms after drinking a usual sized serving of milk (i.e., 8 oz, 237 ml, which contains only 12 g of lactose), and whether such symptoms are of clinical importance.

This concept of "milk intolerance" rather then lactose intolerance is extremely important, since milk is supplied all over the world in school feeding programs and other supplementation programs. A number of studies have demonstrated intolerance to a single glass of milk in children who are lactose intolerant. Symptoms, however, were much milder. A few studies have failed to document any significant symptoms. Hence at present the data are by no means definitive. However, it would appear that enough chidren will exhibit discomfort after consuming a glass of milk to begin to think of supplying alternative sources of protein in school feeding programs. This is particularly important because the relatively high incidence of milk rejection reported from some schools may be due in part to milk intolerance. It should be pointed out, however, that in many countries throughout the world, and in certain populations within our own country, milk supplementation provides a significant proportion of the total protein consumed. Until alternative sources are available such supplementation should be continued in spite of the fact that some children might exhibit some discomfort.

RECOMMENDED READING

Background Information on Lactose and Milk Intolerance, *Nutr. Rev.,* **30,** 175 (1972).

Bayless T. M., and D. M. Paige, Lactose Intolerance, in *Nutritional Management of Genetic Disorders,* M. Winick, Ed., Wiley, New York, 1979, pp. 79–90.

Committee on Nutrition, American Academy of Pediatrics, Should Milk Drinking by Children be Discouraged? *Pediatrics,* **53,** 576 (1974).

Dreizer, S., The Importance of Nutrition in Tooth Development, *J. School Health,* **43,** 114 (1973).

The Etiology and Implications of Lactose Intolerance, *Nutr. Rev.,* **31,** 182 (1973).

Fomon, S. J., *Infant Nutrition,* 2nd ed., Saunders, Philadelphia, 1974.

Grenby, T. H., The Effects of Some Carbohydrates on Experimental Dental Caries in the Rat, *Arch. Oral Biol.,* **8,** 27 (1963).

Grenby, T. H., Dental Plaque Studies on Baboons Fed on Diets Containing Different Carbohydrates, *Arch. Oral Biol.,* **16,** 631 (1971).

Halzel, A. V. Schwartz, and K. W. Sutcliffe, Defective Lactose Absorption Causing Malnutrition in Infancy, *Lancet,* **1,** 1126 (1959).

Hofeldt, F. D., Reactive Hypoglycemia, *Metab.,* **24,** 1973 (1975).

Kuitunen, P., J. Rappola, E. Savilahti, and J. K. Visakorpi, Response of the Jejunal Mucosa to Cow's Milk in the Malabsorption Syndrome with Cow's Milk Intolerance. A Light- and Electron-Microscopic Study, *Acta Paediat. Scandinav.,* **62,** 585 (1973).

Lactose Activity Levels in Nigeria—Genetic or Acquired Phenomenon? *Nutr. Rev.,* **30,** 156 (1972).

Makinen, K. K., and L. Philosophy, The Role of Sucrose and Other Sugars in the Development of Dental Caries, *Int. Dent. J.,* **22,** 363 (1972).

Newbrun, E., Sucrose, The Arch Criminal of Dental Caries, *J. Dent. Child.,* **36,** 239, (1969).

Neale, G., The Geographical Incidence of Lactase Deficiency, *Path. Microbiol.,* **39,** 238 (1973).

Simons, F. J., Progress Report. New Light on Ethnic Differences in Adult Lactose Intolerance, *Am. J. Dig. Dis.,* **18,** 595 (1973).

Statement on Hypoglycemia, *Arch. Int. Med.,* **131,** 591 (1973).

Stephenson, L. S., and M. C. Latham, Lactose Intolerance and Milk Consumption: The Relation of Tolerance to Symptoms, *Am. J. Clin. Nutr.,* **27,** 296 (1974).

15

EXCESS VITAMINS, MINERALS, AND FOOD ADDITIVES

In recent years there has been a tendency for people to consume larger and larger quantities of vitamins and minerals to "prevent disease" or to achieve "optimal health." During the past 25 years a number of vitamins in large doses have been advocated for the treatment of numerous diseases not caused by a specific deficiency of the vitamin in question. For example, certain psychiatric disorders such as schizophrenia have been treated with large doses of thiamin or niacin. More recently a group of people from within the medical profession and from the general public have advocated the use of large doses of vitamins and minerals to "promote optimal health." Since the definition of optimal health is, at best, obscure, it is difficult, if not impossible, to know whether this type of prophylaxis has any benefit at all.

We have noted in Chapter 10 how difficult it has become to set even "normal" vitamin requirements as lifestyles change and people smoke, consume alcohol and drugs, and adopt eating patterns that may reduce intake. When one tries to set requirements for something as nebulous as optimal health the task becomes monumental. However, it is important to continue to think in these terms since certainly our function as physicians is more than just the prevention of overt disease. The problem is that a vitamin or a mineral in very large doses is no longer supplying an essential nutrient in trace amounts. Micronutrients in these doses are pharmacological substances and must be examined in the same way as any therapeutic drug. Efficacy must be determined, toxicity must be assessed, and then a judgment must be rendered whether the therapeutic result is important enough in the face of whatever toxicity may be present. With some vitamins this is easily accomplished; with others, because both efficacy and toxicity are minimal or nondemonstrable, controversy still rages.

Since the fat-soluble vitamins can be stored in the body, effects of excess ingestion are cumulative. Toxicity with these vitamins will occur and clinically significant disease can be produced by excess ingestion, especially of vitamins A and D.

FAT-SOLUBLE VITAMINS

Vitamin A

It is difficult to produce vitamin A toxicity from dietary sources although it has been reported in Eskimos consuming polar bear liver which is an extremely rich source of vitamin A. By contrast, vitamin A intoxication can and does occur in both an acute and a chronic form secondary to the ingestion of large quantities of the vitamin from supplemental sources. Symptoms of acute vitamin A poisoning will occur within a few hours after the ingestion of 75,000 to 300,000 IU in infants and of two million IU in adults. In infants signs of increased intracranial pressure with anorexia, vomiting, hyperirritability, and bulging fontanelles will rapidly develop. In adults, central nervous system symptoms, such as headache, drowsiness, dizziness, and nausea and vomiting, as well as dermatosis, such as erythema and persistent desquamation, may develop.

When more than 10,000 IU/day are consumed, chronic toxicity can develop in children within months, whereas in adults such toxicity usually takes several years to manifest itself. The signs of chronic toxicity in children again develop within the central nervous system but are also manifested by changes in skin and bones. Signs of increased intracranial pressure slowly develop, sutures widen, and fontanelles bulge in young infants, and headache occurs in older children as cerebrospinal fluid pressure increases. Irritability, alternating with periods of lethargy, is often observed. Examination of the eyegrounds reveals what appears to be papilledema, and a syndrome referred to as pseudotumor cerebri will result. Children with this syndrome have sometimes been studied for brain tumors, and some have even been explored. Thus in any child manifesting central nervous system symptoms and signs of increased intracranial pressure for no apparent reason, vitamin A toxicity must be considered. The skin manifestations of chronic toxicity include itching, exfoliative dermatitis, angular stomatitis, and frequent paronychiae. Changes in the bones include hyperostosis and metaphyseal cupping. If the toxicity continues for a long enough time, optic atrophy and blindness may result.

In adults, chronic toxicity affects a number of organ systems. Again central nervous system symptoms predominate, with headache, nausea and vomiting, weakness, and in some cases profound psychiatric symptoms which have led to hospitalization for severe depression or schizophrenia. The changes in skin include dryness, alopecia, and desquamation. Hepatic dysfunction accompanied by hepatosplenomegaly and even ascites has been reported. In certain cases a marked elevation in serum calcium occurs. In addition to these symptoms, nonspecific symptoms, such as pains in the abdomen, muscles, joints, and bones, are reported.

The severe toxicity associated with high doses of vitamin A certainly precludes its use in such doses as a prophylactic agent to prevent disease or to promote optimal health, and even the most ardent supporters of the use of megavitamins exclude vitamin A. Recently, however, based on the skin manifestations induced by high doses of vitamin A, an indirect prophylactic role in certain types of cancer is being explored. The data in animals suggested that high doses of vitamin A offered protection against the induction of certain epithelial tumors (i.e., lung, prostate, bladder). Moreover, the site on the vitamin A molecule producing skin activity was different from the site producing other toxic manifestations, such as those in the central nervous system. Hence by altering the molecule of vitamin A and producing vitamin A analogs, preparations were synthesized which had the same or greater anticancer effects but much less toxicity. This line of research has progressed to the point where analogs have been produced, have been extensively tested in animals, and are now being used in clinical trials. It should be noted that these vitamin A analogs have no effect in curing an already established cancer. Their use is in *preventing* the tumor from being induced by known carcinogens. Hence, the therapeutic trials being organized are in populations at very high risk for developing certain types of carcinoma. For example, people with bladder papillomas that have been removed have a very high incidence of recurrence and eventual malignant transformation. Asbestos plant workers have an extremely high risk for lung cancer. If this approach is successful, as we identify more and more at risk groups, the use of vitamin A analogs in cancer prophylaxis could become important.

Vitamin D

In large doses vitamin D, like vitamin A, is extremely toxic. Again the danger is in cumulative ingestion of high doses, since the vitamin is stored. With vitamin D, the chances for chronic toxicity are greater than with vitamin A, since the margin between amounts necessary to fulfill requirements and amounts capable of producing toxicity is much smaller, especially in children. Some very sensitive children may develop symptoms of toxicity upon ingestion of doses very close to the recommended 400 IU. Since many foods are fortified with vitamin D, children may consume large amounts inadvertently. In fact, a major disaster occurred in Great Britain in the early 1950s when in reaction to wartime deprivation a number of staple foods were fortified with vitamin D. Milk was fortified at a higher than usual amount (800 IU) per quart). The result was an epidemic of what only later was discovered to be vitamin D toxicity. Children were growth retarded at birth, and had elfin facies and high levels of serum calcium. The disease was at first called idiopathic hypercalcemia and was seen at birth or developed during the first year of life. Many of these children developed mental retardation and some progressed to renal failure and death. Eventually, through outstanding investigations by British epidemiologists, the cause of the disease was identified as a form of chronic vitamin D toxicity in susceptible populations. The British responded by reducing the amount of vitamin D used in fortification and the disease has virtually disappeared.

I point to this experience not only as a historical event illustrating the small margin between vitamin D requirements and vitamin D toxicity but because we in the United States are moving closer and closer to the danger zone.

It is far from unusual for an American child to awaken in the morning, take a vitamin pill with 100% of the daily vitamin D requirement, eat a bowl of "fortified" cereal (another 100%) with milk in the cereal, and drink a glass of milk afterwards (another 50% of the daily requirement). Hence, on leaving for school the child has already consumed 250% of the RDA. It is not difficult under these circumstances for four or five times the RDA to be consumed daily.

It is ironic that this situation should be developing with vitamin D, since vitamin D in food represents a reserve system and is necessary only when sunlight is unavailable and precursors in the skin are not being converted. The average child probably does not need any vitamin D, especially in the summer time. And yet vitamin D toxicity is still seen in many places. Besides the symptoms described in young infants, ingestion of 1000 to 2000 IU/day (2.5 to 5 times the RDA) has produced signs of toxicity in children, including growth retardation. In very high amounts (10 times the RDA or more) vitamin D will produce hypercalcemia in adults as well as children. This is associated with weakness, anorexia, vomiting, and diarrhea. Polydipsia, polyuria, and proteinuria may develop if kidney function is compromised, and ectopic calcium deposition may occur in various soft tissues. If vitamin D toxicity continues for a long enough period, renal failure and death may ensue.

As with vitamin A, vitamin D in large amounts is too toxic to be advocated for prophylaxis. Again even the most avid megavitamin enthusiasts do not advocate high doses of vitamin D. And yet with our tendency to fortify foods and to consume multivitamin preparations we are slowly increasing our vitamin D intake to levels that are reason for concern.

Vitamin E

Vitamin E is the one fat-soluble vitamin that is advocated by some in very large doses for the prevention of a variety of conditions. These include the effects of old age, cancer, air pollution damage, skin inflammations, habitual abortions, heart disease, menopausal syndrome, infertility, peptic ulcer, burns, and neuromuscular disorders. In addition, high doses of vitamin E are being marketed as able to increase both male and female sexual potency. There is no clinical evidence to support any of these claims, and even the animal evidence upon which some of the claims are supposedly based has been distorted. Only anecdotal evidence exists that vitamin E in large doses has any therapeutic value. From the standpoint of toxicity, vitamin E is obviously different from vitamins A and D. Although it is stored in the body, serious toxic reactions have rarely been reported even after ingestion of large amounts, although certain nonspecific symptoms have been reported in some patients. These have promptly disappeared when vitamin E was discontinued. This situation has resulted in the argument that since no real toxicity has been demonstrated, there is no danger in large doses and hence why not take them just to be on the safe side. This argument is extremely dangerous with any agent—surely it would not be accepted for a drug or an air pollutant or a food additive—and yet because the agent being advocated is a vitamin, many people accept it. The argument is especially dangerous when the agent, in this case vitamin E, is stored within the body. If we have learned anything during the past few years in relation to nutrition and health, it has been that the effects of nutrient excess may take many years to manifest themselves. Atherosclerosis may begin in infancy and culminate at age 70 in a coronary infarction. Cancer may develop in old age after lifelong exposure to certain nutritional excesses. The long-term toxicity of chronic ingestion of high doses of vitamin E could take several more decades before it is recognized. Hence only if there is a specific proven therapeutic benefit to large doses should they be used. Since no such benefit has yet been demonstrated, I cannot recommend the use of high doses of vitamin E. However, as further research is conducted, high doses of vitamin E may prove to be useful in the treatment of some conditions. At that point, relative risk versus efficacy would have to be evaluated. One such condition may be intermittent claudication, which in some cases has been reported to respond to high doses of vitamin E. Since this is a serious and debilitating problem when it occurs, a therapeutic trial of vitamin E may be undertaken.

WATER-SOLUBLE VITAMINS

Excess ingestion of water-soluble vitamins presents a different problem from excess ingestion of fat-soluble vitamins. Because they are not stored in the body, they do not accumulate in tissues to any great extent and hence the danger of cumulative long-term toxicity is much less. However, the fact that the excess is rapidly excreted may in itself present a problem, in that large doses of the vitamin may be excreted in urine and may have specific effects of the kidney and organs of the urinary tract. There is some evidence that this is the case with vitamin C. At least one of the water-soluble vitamins in high doses, niacin or nicotinic acid, will produce symptoms such as hyperemia, flushing of the face and extremities, and palpitations. In fact, this agent had been used in the past to treat certain forms of vascular disease. The other vitamins, as far as we know, do not produce any acute symptoms even in very large doses.

Many of the water-soluble vitamins have been used to treat a variety of illnesses throughout this century. The illnesses treated have been mainly those whose symptoms are in some way similar to symptoms of deficiency of the particular vitamin. Thus, because thiamin deficiency is associated with central nervous system changes, thiamin has been advocated in large doses for the treatment of mental illnesses ranging from schizophrenia and other psychoses to mental retardation. There are no controlled studies to support the efficacy of such treatment and gradually, through the years, one form of vitamin therapy has been replaced with yet another vitamin or combination of vitamins. It should be noted that in most cases the diseases being treated were serious and were or are not amenable to any other known treatment. Hence the vitamin therapy was being used as a desperate measure. There is little to criticize in this approach as long as the physician remains objective and as long as the use of such therapy in no way compromises the use of other available therapy which may control, and in some cases even cure, the disease. Unfortunately, however, new vitamins have sometimes been invented for the purpose of treating certain serious diseases, as is currently the case in the area of cancer treatment, where laetrile, hailed by its proponents as vitamin B_{17}, is being used in therapy. Certainly this agent is not a vitamin, since it is not essential for any known function and since its complete absence in the diet causes no known abnormalities. No controlled studies have demonstrated any efficacy of this substance in the treatment of cancer. Moreover, it is obviously toxic to some extent, since it contains cyanide, a deadly poison. Finally, however, it is most dangerous because it is sometimes used *instead* of conventional therapy, which in the early stages might control or cure the disease. Recently, certain states have banned the sale of laetrile within their borders. This has come about because of the use of this substance by so-called health professionals. Certainly, there is no reason to undertake this kind of treatment based on present knowledge.

Vitamin C

The vitamin for which the best case has been made for the use of considerably larger amounts than have been recommended is vitamin C, or ascorbic acid. The data are certainly not all in at present; however, it is useful to examine available data to see whether tentative recommendations can be made.

Only small amounts of ascorbic acid (10 to 20 mg/day) are necessary to prevent scurvy. Slightly more is necessary to cure scurvy. Why then are some people advocating 1 g/day or more? The argument is based on extrapolations from other animals who require vitamin C, for example, the guinea pig, who on a weight basis would require this amount, and on the usual amounts consumed by other ascorbic acid requiring mammals, for example, fruit bats and subhuman primates. From these data some proponents of higher doses of vitamin C argue that the RDA has been set much too low and that the higher doses they recommend are, in fact, the physiological requirement which man, because of a gradual change in lifestyle and eating patterns, no longer gets from his food. By contrast, those who have set the present requirement base their recommendations on blood and tissue saturation levels. They cite several studies which demonstrate that at the recommended level (40 mg/day), blood levels are high and tissues, such as leukocytes, are saturated. While neither type of data is definitive, the explanation based on comparative studies does not take into account species variation and the fact that even animals that require vitamin C show differences in ascorbic acid metabolism. Moreover, even if we reverted to an entirely agrarian lifestyle, it would be extremely difficult to ingest the amount of vitamin C that they recommend from our food supply, especially in northern climates. It should be noted, however, that different tissues might require different amounts of ascorbic acid for saturation, and data limited to certain tissues might have to be revised.

Certainly, the requirement as currently set is not the final answer but as far as we can tell it is in the right range.

The second argument of the proponents of high doses of vitamin C is that in such doses certain prophylactic and therapeutic benefits are manifest. Thus, regardless of what the actual requirement might be, high doses protect against such illnesses as the common cold, nonspecific stress, and cancer. The only reasonably controlled studies in this regard have to do with the common cold. In two studies carried out in Canada by the same group, the results were not conclusive. The first study showed some reduction in the incidence of the common cold in subjects who were given 1 g/day of vitamin C prophylactically, and some shortening of symptoms when 4 g/day were used in treatment. The second study showed no effect. At best, then, doses of ascorbic acid of 1 g or more have only a slight effect on the incidence or severity of the common cold. Thus, efficacy is minimal. What about toxicity? Large doses increase the amount excreted in urine, since vitamin C is not stored to any appreciable extent. This results in acidification of the urine. Whether this might affect the urinary tract and bladder over long periods is unknown.

Recently, another side effect of prolonged high doses has been reported in pregnant guinea pigs and is suspected in pregnant women. Guinea pigs exposed to high doses of ascorbic acid during pregnancy give birth to pups who develop scurvy more rapidly when reared without additional vitamin C. This occurs because vitamin C is catabolized more rapidly in these pups and hence reserves are used up faster. Thus a sort of vitamin C dependency syndrome has developed which will disappear after a time on smaller amounts of vitamin C. Several cases of scurvy have been reported in human infants born to mothers who consume large doses of vitamin C, and in adults maintained on high levels of vitamin C, when the vitamin is withdrawn blood levels of ascorbic acid drop to a greater degree than in individuals maintained on lower levels. Again, these data suggest a transient dependency due to the induction of a mechanism that increases catabolism of ascorbic acid.

The data, then, suggest that some undesirable side effects can be induced by prolonged use of high doses of ascorbic acid. On balance, although I am not convinced that the RDA of 40 mg/day is high enough, I feel that doses of 1 g and above are certainly outside the physiological range. Hence, vitamin C in these doses, like any agent consumed in nonphysiological amounts, must be considered in the same way as one considers a drug. Efficacy must first be proven. This has not yet been done to my satisfaction. When there is in addition even potential toxicity, I must advise restraint. Hence, at present, I cannot advocate the use of high doses of vitamin C in prophylaxis.

EXCESS MINERALS

At least two minerals are consumed by many people in their normal diets in amounts that are far above what is necessary and may even be detrimental to health. These are sodium and phosphorus. Other minerals, like many vitamins, are being recommended as supplements in high doses to protect against nonspecific disease, such as iron for fatigue, or zinc, copper, and magnesium for "deficiency states" which do not exist. The excess consumption of sodium and phosphorus is the more serious problem, since it may be contributing to two very common and very serious diseases, hypertension and osteoporosis. Although the data are not conclusive, the evidence suggests that our high sodium intake, especially when coupled with our relatively low potassium intake, materially contributes to the high incidence of hypertension in many developed countries. Similar evidence, although not as compelling as that for sodium and potassium, suggests that our high phosphorus intake, especially when coupled with a low calcium intake, contributes to the high incidence of osteoporosis in our middle aged and elderly populations.

Sodium

Many studies indicate that sodium chloride will increase blood pressure in most hypertensives. Moreover most patients with essential hypertension who respond to diuretic drugs will respond equally well to dietary sodium restriction. Most physicians, however, prefer the use of diuretics, in patients with good renal function, because of the difficulty in our society of maintaining a patient on a sodium intake of around 500 mg/day (slightly more than 1 g of NaCl).

The average daily requirement for sodium is of the order of a few hundred milligrams per day, probably no more than half a gram. Even the recommended allowance of 1 g/day of NaCl per liter of water intake as liquid and food, which is certainly high, would suggest less than 3 g/day of sodium chloride in most people. The actual average intake in our society is between 6 and 18 g. Thus we consume two to six times what is recommended and perhaps 10 to 35 times what is actually needed. On the other hand, the intake of potassium in our society is undoubtedly much less than optimal.

There are a number of reasons for this high sodium, low potassium environment not the least of which is the fact that much of our food is processed and that processing often increases sodium content and decreases potassium content. Table 1 is an example of the changes undergone by 100 g of peas under certain processing conditions. Thus the canned peas drained of fluid contain 255 times as much sodium as the fresh peas before

Table 1. Changes in sodium and potassium content of peas

Food (100 g Edible Portion)	Na (mg)	K (mg)
Fresh peas	0.9	380
Frozen peas	100	160
Canned peas (liquid poured off)	230	180

salted butter and added salt are used. In addition, more than half the potassium is gone. Although this does not happen to all food in processing, it is not unusual. Table 2 shows the sodium and potassium content of a number of common processed foods. At present, with consumption of table salt declining, sodium intake is determined more by the food processors than by the individual.

Recently, the Committee on Nutrition of the American Academy of Pediatrics concluded that the intake of salt by young infants was several times what was needed. They recommended reducing the salt content of baby foods. Since this recommendation, most baby food manufacturers have stopped adding salt to their proucts. When the child changes to table food, however, there is a marked increase in NaCl intake.

Table 2. Sodium and potassium content of several processed foods

Food (100 g Edible Portion)	Na (mg)	K (mg)
Olives	2400	55
White bread	507	105
Cornflakes	660	160
Cheddar cheese	700	82
Dried nonfat milk	525	1335
Bacon	1770	225
Chipped beef	4300	200
Smoked ham, raw	2530	248
Frankfurter	1100	230
Salami	1260	302
Canned crab meat	1000	110
Canned salmon	540	330

What is the evidence that this high sodium, low potassium environment is contributing to the problem of hypertension in our society?

Animal experiments have demonstrated that certain rat strains will develop hypertension when placed on a high sodium diet alone. Other strains will develop hypertension when placed on a high sodium, low potassium diet. Since these effects occur only in particular strains, the propensity for sodium-induced hypertension clearly has a genetic component. Hence, as with many other nutritional factors, there is an interplay between environmental and genetic factors in the genesis of the disease process.

Hypertension in humans also has a genetic component. It is much more common among certain racial groups. For example, it is more common among blacks than whites. It is estimated that 20% of the adult population in the United States has elevated blood pressure. Among blacks this number may be as high as 50%. Most individuals who have high blood pressure with no organic cause (essential hypertension) will respond to salt restriction or salt excretion induced by diuretic agents. Finally, in countries where the intake of salt is low, even susceptible populations such as blacks show a much lower incidence of hypertension.

It has been said that our high salt intake is in part a physiological response, in that all animals, including the human, crave salt. Controlled experiments have demonstrated that on the contrary salt preference is learned rather than innate.

What, then, can we do about this problem? Certainly the food industry should be encouraged to lower the sodium content of processed foods whenever possible. Susceptible populations, such as blacks and any other people with a family history of hypertension, should be urged to lower their salt intake, and when possible, to consume foods low in sodium and high in potassium. These people might be encouraged to use sodium-potassium chloride as a complete replacement for sodium chloride. This will allow similar flavoring while materially reducing sodium intake and increasing potassium intake. If these measures could be successfully accomplished we would expect a significant reduction in the incidence of high blood pressure within our society. This, in turn, would significantly reduce mortality and morbidity from coronary artery disease and stroke, two of the major killers of modern society.

Phosphorus

The second mineral undoubtedly consumed in excess amounts by the general population is phosphorus. Certainly phosphorus is an essential element. Although its deficiency state can be experimentally produced, it occurs in humans only as an accompaniment to serious disease, usually involving the kidney or the parathyroid gland. By contrast, excess phosphorus is consumed by most people, often beginning at birth, and may contribute to certain disease processes. It has been clearly demonstrated that calcium absorption depends in part on the amount of phosphorus in the diet (see Chapter 10). Calcium:phosphorus ratios of lower than 2:1 enhance bone resorption. Dietary phosphorus in many human diets is two to four times greater than calcium content, depending on the nature of the food supply. As with sodium and potassium, we live in a high phosphorus, low calcium environment.

This high phosphorus environment begins at birth if the infant is fed a cow's milk formula. While human milk contains 150 to 175 mg/liter of phosphorus, cow's milk contains about 1000 mg/liter. Even when suitably diluted to equalize the protein content, a formula made from cow's milk will contain three times as much phosphorus as human milk. There is some evidence that this may contribute to hypocalcemic tetany, which may occur during the first weeks of life in infants fed cow's milk formulas.

In adults the consumption of large amounts of meat coupled with the intake of numerous carbonated drinks and other foods high in phosphorus has increased our phosphorus intake markedly during the past century.

The data relating high phosphorus and relatively low calcium intake to osteoporosis are at present only suggestive. There is no question that the kind of calcium:phosphorus ratio consumed by many people will promote bone resorption in both animals and humans. Whether such bone resorption over a long period of time contributes to the problem of osteoporosis in the elderly is not yet determined. The evidence is suggestive enough, however, for us to encourage reduction in phosphorus intakes.

Trace Minerals

The trace minerals are present in our food supply in small amounts and hence excess of trace minerals does not occur under ordinary conditions. However, there has been a trend to "prophylactic" use of megadoses of certain minerals. While this practice is by no means as common as with vitamins, it too is potentially dangerous. Large doses of certain essential minerals are known to be toxic. For example, both acute and chronic iron poisoning can occur. The chronic form, caused by cumulative intake of high doses, will result in hemosiderosis with deposits of hemosiderin in many tissues. We do not know what chronic administration of high doses of such minerals as zinc, chromium, and so forth would result in, but since there is no reason for using high doses of minerals the practice should be discouraged.

FOOD ADDITIVES

A detailed discussion of food additives is beyond the scope of this book and fits better into a discussion of toxicology. However, since certain claims are being made about the relation of food additives to health some comments are in order.

Additives are added to our foods for a number of reasons, such as to enhance color, odor, or flavor, or for the preservation of freshness. The first three are more or less cosmetic; the last is necessary if we are to maintain the type of food distribution system that most developed countries have. Hence we cannot lump all food additives together; nor should our food additive laws do this. And yet they seem to.

At present the Food and Drug Administration requires a number of tests before an additive can be used. However, this array is the same no matter what the purpose of the additive. By law (Delaney Law) any food additive that causes cancer in any dose in any laboratory animal must be removed from the food supply. It is this law that has led to the removal of such agents as red dye II and saccharin. There are some who feel that the law is too rigid in that some agents would have to be consumed in enormous amounts to reproduce the conditions that resulted in tumors under the experimental conditions. My own view is that the law is all right for additives affecting only color, flavor, or odor, but that it is too rigid for additives that are protecting the safety of our food supply or offering some other health benefit.

Recently there have been claims that food additives may be contributing to hyperactivity (hyperkinesis) in children. Although the data were mostly anecdotal, the problem is severe enough to have created a major controversy in pediatric circles. The few controlled studies that have been done suggest that most children, especially those over 3 years, will not respond objectively to diets that eliminate all additives. Some children (all under 3 years) do respond. Thus in children under 3 with hyperkinesis, a diet free of food additives might be tried. If no change occurs, the child should not be kept on this diet, since it is difficult to adhere to and it singles the child out as being different when this is not necessary.

The widespread use of food additives has no doubt made our food supply safer and more attractive. However, like anything else, the practice can be abused. At present the public is concerned, and rightly so, that this might be happening. It is important that a strong system be initiated and maintained to protect the public interest in this very sensitive area.

RECOMMENDED READING

Vitamins

Anderson, T. W., D. B. Reid, and G. H. Beaton. Vitamin C and the Common Cold: A Double Blind Trial, *Canad. Med. J.,* **107,** 503 (1972).

Ascorbic Acid and the Common Cold, *Nutr. Rev.,* **25,** 684 (1972).

Bieri, J. G., Effect of Excessive Vitamin C and E on Vitamin A Status, *Am. J. Clin. Nutr.,* **26,** 382 (1973).

Canadian Pediatric Society, The Use and Abuse of Vitamin A, *Canad. Med. J.,* **104,** 521 (1971).

Committee on Nutrition, American Academy of Pediatrics, The Prophylactic Requirement and Toxicity of Vitamin D, *Pediatrics,* **31,** 512 (1963).

Committee on Nutrition, American Academy of Pediatrics, Vitamin D Intake and the Hypercalcemic Syndrome, *Pediatrics,* **35,** 1022 (1965).

Coulehan, J. L., K. S. Reisinger, K. D. Rogers, and D. W. Bradley, Vitamin C Prophylaxis in a Boarding School, *N. Engl. J. Med.,* **290,** 6 (1974).

Di Benedetto, R. J., Chronic Hypervitaminosis A in an Adult, *J.A.M.A.,* **201,** 130 (1967).

Favus, M. J., Treatment of Vitamin D Intoxication, *New Engl. J. Med.,* **283,** 1468 (1970).

Frimpter, G. W., K. J. Andelman, and W. F. George, Vitamin B_6 Dependency Syndromes: New Horizons in Nutrition, *Am. J. Clin. Nutr.,* **22,** 794 (1969).

Hazards of Overdose of Vitamin D, *Nutr. Rev.,* **33,** 61 (1975).

Katz, C. M., and M. Tzagournis, Chronic Adult Hypervitaminosis A with Hypercalcemia, *Metab.,* **21,** 1171 (1972).

Mayer, J., Vitamins and Mental Disorders, *Postgrad. Med.,* **45,** 268 (1969).

Muenter, M. D., H. O. Perry, and J. Ludwig, Chronic Vitamin A Intoxication in Adults, *Am. J. Med.,* **50,** 129 (1971).

Norkus, E., and P. Rosso, Oral Contraceptives and Vitamin B_6, *Nutr. Rev.,* **31,** 49 (1973).

Pelletier, O., Vitamin C Status of Cigarette Smokers and Non-Smokers, *Am. J. Clin. Nutr.,* **23,** 520 (1970).

Roe, D. A., Nutrient Toxicity with Excessive Intake, I Vitamins, *N.Y. State J. Med.,* **66,** 869 (1966).

Sezlig, M. S., Vitamin D and Cardiovascular Renal and Brain Damage in Infancy and Childhood, *Ann., N.Y. Acad. Sci.,* **147,** 537 (1969).

Supplementation of Human Diets with Vitamin E., *Nutr. Rev.,* **30,** 327 (1973).

Vitamin A Intoxication in Infancy, *Nutr. Rev.,* **23,** 265 (1965).

Vitamin E, Miracle or Myth? *FDA Consumer,* **7,** 24 (1973).

Minerals

Adlin, E. V., C. M. Biddle, and B. J. Channie, Dietary Salt Intake in Hypertensive Patients with Normal and Low Plasma Renin Activity, *Am. J. Med. Sci.,* **261,** 67 (1974).

Brown, W. J., Jr., F. K. Brown, and I. Krishan, Exchangeable Sodium and Blood Volume in Normotensive and Hypertensive Humans on High and Low Sodium Intake, *Circulation,* **43,** 508 (1971).

Committee on Nutrition, American Academy of Pediatrics, Salt Intake and Eating Patterns of Infants and Children in Relation to Blood Pressure, *Pediatrics,* 53, 115 (1974).

Dahl, L. K., Salt and Hypertension. *Am. J. Clin. Nutr.,* 25, 231 (1972).

Edmondson, R. P. S., R. D. Thomas, P. J. Hilton, and J. Patrick, Abnormal Leucocyte Composition and Sodium Transport in Essential Hypertension, *Lancet,* 1, 1003 (1975).

Gros, G., J. M. Weller, and S. W. Hoobler, Relationship of Sodium and Potassium Intake to Blood Pressure, *Am. J. Clin. Nutr.,* 24, 605 (1971).

Meneely, G. R., C. O. T. Ball, and J. B. Youmans, Chronic Sodium Chloride Toxicity: The Protective Effect of Added Potassium Chloride, *Ann. Int. Med.,* 47, 263 (1957).

Meneely, G. R., and C. O. T. Ball, Experimental Epidemiology of Chronic Sodium Chloride Toxicity and the Protective Effect of Potassium Chloride, *Am. J. Med.,* 25, 713 (1958).

Meneely, G. R., and C. O. T. Ball, in *Hypertension Mineral Metabolism,* Volume VI, American Heart Association, New York, 1958, pp. 65–87.

Meneely, G. R., and L. K. Dahl, Electrolytes in Hypertension: The Effects of Sodium Treatment, *Med. Clin. N. Am.,* 45, 271 (1961).

McDonough, J., and C. M. Wilhelmj, The Effect of Excessive Salt Intake on Human Blood Pressure, *Am. J. Digest. Dis.,* 21, 180 (1954).

Smirk, F. H., in *The Epidemiology of Hypertension,* J. Stamier, R. Stamier, and T. N. Pullman, Eds., Grune and Stratton, New York, 1967, pp. 39–55.

Tobian, L., M. Ishii and M. Duke, Relationship of Cytoplasmic Granules in Renal Papillary Interstitial Cells to "Post-Salt Hypertension," *J. Lab. Clin. Med.,* 73, 309 (1969).

16

EXCESS ALCOHOL

Perhaps the most unrecognized nutritional excess in the United States and in many developed and developing countries is the ingestion of excess alcohol. There are several levels on which alcohol relates to nutrition. Alcoholic beverages themselves are nutrients which provide mostly calories. They may displace essential nutrients in the diet. They can affect appetite and hence food intake. They can alter the metabolism of specific nutrients. Through the direct toxic effects of alcohol, metabolism may be altered and hence nutritional requirements may change. Finally, as a result of the specific effects of alcohol on the liver, which plays a central role in the metabolism of many important nutrients, nutrient metabolism may be deranged.

Based on average national consumption figures, alcohol contributes about 5% of the calories in the American diet. However, in the heavy drinker it is estimated to supply up to 50% of the total calories.

Except for some differences in carbohydrate content and in the levels of some vitamins and minerals, the major nutrient in alcoholic beverages is calories derived from ethanol. Although ethanol liberates 7.1 cal/g, the caloric food value of ethanol is less than that of an isocaloric equivalent of carbohydrate. Thus substituting isocaloric amounts of ethanol for carbohydrate will result in weight loss. Moreover, when given as additional calories, ethanol causes less weight gain than calorically equivalent carbohydrate. Although the mechanism by which this reduced caloric effect takes place is not entirely known, the evidence points to an increased metabolic rate. For example, oxygen consumption increases in normal people when ethanol is ingested and this increase is even greater in alcoholics. Hence alcoholic beverages provide little nutritive value other than calories, and the calories are not utilized as well as in equivalent amounts in carbohydrate.

Although in general the stereotype of the typical alcoholic as an emaciated severely undernourished individual is no longer true, certainly severe alcoholism, even in higher socioeconomic groups, can result in moderate and sometimes severe malnutrition. This may be due to reduced food intake resulting from reduced appetite, chronic gastritis, or depressed consciousness.

The major nutritional consequences of excess alcohol are due to its direct toxic effects, especially on the liver. As a result of chronic ingestion of large amounts of alcohol, fatty liver, hepatitis, and cirrhosis can occur. Although the most serious complications, such as encephalopathy or ascites, usually occur in patients with cirrhosis, they have been well documented in the presence of fatty liver alone.

A second organ system on which ethanol exhibits direct toxicity is the gastrointestinal tract. Ethanol can effect gastric acid secretion and gastric emptying time and is an accepted cause of acute gastritis. It is directly injurious to the mucosa of the small intestines, and impaired absorption of fat, xylose, folate, thiamin, and B_{12} have been described in the chronic alcoholic. In acute alcoholic toxicity the absorption of many other nutrients may also be impaired. Pancreatic secretions can be altered in chronic alcoholism and both acute and chronic pancreatitis are associated with alcoholism. Bile salts may also be reduced in the alcoholic. All of these changes in the gastrointestinal tract may lead to a malabsorption syndrome.

Besides affecting certain organ systems which are important in maintaining proper nutrition, alcohol exerts direct effects on the metabolism of certain nutrients.

When ethanol is given as isocaloric replacement for carbohydrate, protein breakdown is stimulated and urea content in urine increases. Alcohol has also been reported to alter amino acid metabolism in the liver. Experimental administration of a single large dose of alcohol may inhibit protein synthesis.

Glucose homeostasis is impaired in alcoholic liver disease. Fasting hypoglycemia and impaired glucose tolerance following heavy drinking have been reported. Elevated insulin levels and abnormal glucagon responses have been described in patients with alcoholic cirrhosis.

Lipid metabolism depends in part on normal liver function and may be abnormal in the alcoholic. Increased hepatic ketogenesis, decreased fatty acid oxidation, and increased fatty acid synthesis may lead to an increase in triglycerides which may either accumulate in the liver or be liberated into the blood.

Characteristically chronic alcohol consumption increases all of the lipo-protein fractions in serum. Almost any of the different types of hyper-lipidemia (type IV, V, II) can be induced by alcohol. In some patients, particularly those with type IV familial hyperlipidemia, or carbohydrate-induced hyperlipidemia, there is extreme sensitivity to alcohol, and marked elevations of serum lipids may occur with only moderate intake of alcohol.

The consumption of alcohol may impair vitamin metabolism at many levels. Vitamin intake may be reduced as a result of poor diet or anorexia. Absorption may be impaired because of the effects on the gastrointestinal tract. Hepatic stores, particularly of folate, B_6, B_{12}, and niacin, may be depleted. In addition, the utilization of certain vitamins has been reported to be impaired. Particularly important in this respect are folate, thiamin, and pyridoxine. There is evidence that increased hydrolysis of pyridoxal phosphate takes place in the liver of alcoholics, resulting in deactivation of the vitamin.

Circulating levels of pyridoxine and folate are commonly low in chronic alcoholics, especially if they are somewhat malnourished as well. Serum levels of other vitamins, such as thiamin, may also be low in chronic alcoholics. Clinically, megaloblastic anemia due to folate deficiency and neurologic symptoms due to thiamin deficiency are most common. Recently there has been increasing concern about the consumption of alcohol during pregnancy. Several studies have shown that heavy alcohol intake during the first trimester is associated with an increase in congenital malformations. Moreover, there are some data which suggest that even moderate consumption may have undesirable effects on the fetus. This is especially true if moderate malnutrition accompanies the alcoholism.

The first principle of therapy for any type of alcoholic, particularly one manifesting evidence of liver disease, is removal of the offending agent. This, of course, may be extremely difficult in view of the addictive properties of alcohol. If the patient has evidence of fatty liver and no other complications, abstinence and a regular diet will usually effect reversal of the pathologic changes. In patients with alcoholic hepatitis specific therapy may be necessary when they are acutely ill with fever, nausea, vomiting, and encephalopathy. Fluid and electrolyte replacement is essential. Calories should be administered in the intravenous fluids in the form of dextrose. Hypokalemia should be prevented and 50 to 100 mg of thiamine plus several times the daily requirement for the B vitamins (except folate and B_{12}) as well as vitamin C should be administered.

Once oral feedings are possible adequate calories must be supplied. This is accomplished by feeding carbohydrate and fat to a level of 1600 to 2600 cal/day. Protein intake should be adequate to prevent nitrogen wasting but not excessive, to avoid hepatic coma. Initially 0.5 g/kg/day of high quality protein may be tried (30 to 35 g/day). This can be gradually increased over a period of several weeks until about 70 g/day is reached. The administration of amino acids parenterally entails the risk of precipitating hepatic coma and should be used only when oral protein intake is impossible. Oral vitamin B complex should be given, usually in doses of five times the recommended daily allowance. Vitamin K may be administered intramuscularly (10 mg/day for 3 days). In the initial stages of oral feeding small frequent meals are often better tolerated than larger ones.

In the patient with cirrhosis dietary management is similar to the management of hepatitis. However, even greater vigilance must be maintained for associated problems, such as encephalopathy, salt and water retention, renal failure, jaundice, and specific nutrient deficiencies.

RECOMMENDED READING

Bebb, H. T., H. B. Houser, J. C. Witschi, A. S. Littell, and R. K. Fuller, Calorie and Nutrient Contribution of Alcoholic Beverages to the Usual Diets of 155 Adults, *Am. J. Clin. Nutr.*, **24**, 1042 (1971).

Eichner, E. R., and R. J. Hillman, The Evolution of Anemia in Alcoholic Patients, *Am. J. Med.*, **50**, 218 (1971).

Gabuzda, G. J., Nutrition and Liver Disease, *Med. Clin. North Am.*, **54**, 1455 (1970).

Kissin, B., and H. Begletier, Eds., *Biology of Alcoholism*, Plenum, New York, 1974.

Lieber, C. S., L. M. De Carli, and E. Rubin, Sequential Production of Fatty Liver, Hepatitis and Cirrhosis in Sub-human Primates Fed Alcohol with Adequate Diets, *Proc. Natl. Acad. Sci. USA*, **72**, 437 (1975).

Lieber, C. S., and E. Rubin, Alcoholic Fatty Liver, *N. Engl. J. Med.*, **280**, 705 (1969).

Lindenbaum, J., and C. S. Lieber, Effects of Chronic Ethanol Administration on Intestinal Absorption in Man in the Absence of Nutritional Deficiency, *Ann. N.Y. Acad. Sci.* (1975).

Olson, R. E., Nutrition and Alcoholism, in M. G. Wohl and R. S. Goodhart, Eds., *Modern Nutrition in Health and Disease*, Lea and Febiger, Philadelphia, 1964.

Schenker, S., K. J. Brzen, and A. M. Hoyumpa, Hepatic Encephalopathy: Current Status, *Gastroenterology*, **66**, 121 (1974).

Shaw, S., and C. S. Lieber, Alcoholism, in H. A. Schneider, C. E. Anderson, and D. B. Coursin, Eds., *Nutritional Support of Medical Practice*, Harper and Row, Hagerstown, Md., 1977, pp. 202-221.

PART IV

THE USE OF DIETS IN PREVENTION AND TREATMENT

17

DIETS FOR THE
GENERAL PUBLIC

THE TYPICAL WESTERN DIET

The typical western diet is high in calories and relatively high in total and saturated fat, cholesterol, protein, refined carbohydrate, phosphates, and sodium, and low in unrefined carbohydrates and fiber. In recent years this pattern of food consumption has come under more and more criticism.

Let us examine this diet in light of the nutritional considerations discussed in the first three parts of this book and attempt to determine whether we as health professionals can recommend the establishment of eating patterns, acceptable within our culture, which will promote better health than the eating patterns currently in vogue.

There is little question that the total number of calories from all sources, especially when one includes alcohol, is too high in the United States and most of the western world. Caloric excess is probably the worst feature of the American diet. Therefore, Americans should consume less food of all types, particularly foods of high caloric density. How much should total energy intake be curtailed? Since excess ingestion of calories is a relative matter, defined as more calories consumed than expended, the expenditure side of the equation is also important. However, in our relatively sedentary society, we should not be carried away with exercise alone as a means of solving the problem. The input side is overwhelming, and therefore simply increasing exercise, although it helps somewhat, will not balance the equation. If the individual is extremely sedentary, the introduction of a regimen of moderate exercise will not only help expend calories, but may offer some protection against coronary artery disease. The major impact on caloric balance must be achieved in most people by limiting the size of portions consumed and the quality of the individual foods ingested. In general, from the standpoint of calories it is better in our society to err on the side of too little than too much. From a practical standpoint this means some reduction in portion size, but more important is the substitution within meals of foods that are high in bulk but low in calories for those low in bulk but high in calories. Obviously, a portion of celery has markedly fewer calories than an equal amount, by weight, of chocolate mousse. Just as obviously, however, chocolate mousse tastes better. The idea is not to eliminate altogether the chocolate mousses in our diet but to reduce their quantity and replace it with an equal amount in grams of foods that contain many fewer calories. Foods containing fats are calorically extremely dense, and especially when they are sweetened with sugar to make them attractive to the palate, they can be easily consumed in large quantities. Although there is some evidence that the appetite center is controlled partially by total caloric intake, there is also evidence that this control is easily overridden. Thus ingestion of a high fat diet often (although not always) is associated with ingestion of a diet that is high in calories. For this reason alone reduction in the amount of total dietary fat could have a major health benefit. In addition there is some evidence, although it is not yet conclusive, which suggests that ingestion of large amounts of fat from any source over many years is associated with an increased incidence of cancer of the colon and breast (Chapter 13). Since the major source of dietary fat in the typical western diet comes from animal sources, and since it is animal or saturated fat that is associated with coronary artery disease, the number one killer disease in our society, it makes sense to attempt to achieve this reduction by concentrating on saturated fat. As the consumption of saturated fat in our diet is reduced, the ratio of poly-unsaturated to saturated fat (P:S) will increase. It should be noted, however, that simply replacing all of the saturated fat in our diet with unsaturated fat will have no impact on our overconsumption of calories and, as far as we can tell now, little impact on the incidence of cancer of the colon or breast.

Increasing the intake of complex carbohydrates, especially those high in dietary fiber, offers an excellent practical method for substituting an essentially low caloric density food for a high one, and in my judgement this should be the primary way of replacing the fat in our diet while still providing adequate bulk. Such a replacement will automatically reduce the amount of protein in the diet, since much of our fat is consumed in conjunction with protein in the form of meat and meat products. There is no danger in such a reduction, since western society, and particularly Americans, consume too much protein. The reduction in protein itself will also reduce calories somewhat, because the protein component of meat and meat products yields higher amounts of *available* calories than the amount that is derived from an equal weight of complex carbohydrate, much of which is indigestible. In addition, reducing the amount of meat will reduce the quantity of phosphorus in our diet, and this reduction, coupled with the reduced protein, will result in a more positive calcium balance, an added benefit. Finally, as pointed out in Chapter 11, there are certain specific health advantages to increasing the amount of fiber in our diet, in addition to its extremely low caloric density.

As pointed out in Chapter 14, it is not yet clear whether the relatively large amounts of refined sugar consumed by Americans (and even more by certain Europeans) is a significant health problem. A reduction in the amount of refined sugar consumed might have an impact on dental caries, although the magnitude of that impact is by no means clear. Certainly at present fluoridation offers a much more reliable means of control. If the reduction of dental caries is the major health benefit to be derived from decreasing the intake of refined sugar, then concentrating on the form of the sugar and the manner in which it is consumed is probably more important than limiting its total quantity. As pointed out in Chapter 14, there is very little convincing evidence that sugar per se is a major contributor to any other serious health problem except as a source of pleasant, low density calories. To me, then, the sugar used to sweeten fat is most dangerous and would, of course, be reduced if fat consumption were considerably reduced. I am aware that claims have been made that the high consumption of refined sugar beyond the caloric content contributes significantly to coronary artery disease, diabetes, obesity, hypoglycemia, hyperkinesis, and many other diseases. To me, none of the evidence presented by proponents of these theories is convincing. This is not to say that we should not reduce the amount of sugar that we ingest. Sugar contains 4 cal/g, and hence eliminating 5 g of sugar from a cup of coffee can reduce caloric intake by 200 g/day in the heavy coffee drinkers. What I am saying is that beyond portion control the only way to reduce our calories is to alter the quality of our diet by consuming larger amounts of low caloric density foods. These should be used in place of higher caloric density foods. Although refined sugar is higher in caloric density than complex carbohydrates containing large amounts of fiber, fats are more than twice as calorically dense. Hence fat replacement becomes the first priority. Only after this is accomplished and only if caloric intake is still too high should there be public health measures to reduce sugar consumption.

Obviously in any individual case where sugar consumption is high and fat consumption relatively low, if caloric reduction is desirable sugar should be replaced.

Alcohol is an often overlooked source of calories in our diet. One cubic centimeter of absolute alcohol contains 7 cal. Thus hard liquor would contain approximately 3 cal/cc. When one considers the calories in the mixer, even the moderate drinker can be receiving significant calories over the course of a day. With the incidence of heavy drinking as high as it is, in many individuals this can be a major cause of caloric excess quite apart from all of the other nutritional and direct toxic effects of alcohol.

As we have seen in Chapter 15, the sodium content of our diet is extremely high and there is evidence that this sodium excess in certain susceptible individuals is contributing to the extremely high incidence of hypertension in the United States. Much of the sodium in our food supply is added in processing and therefore reaches us often without our knowledge. While rational guidelines have been set, these are often hard to meet. Certainly Americans should be made aware of the problem so that steps to reduce salt intake can be taken.

In summary, the western diet and particularly the American diet could be altered to promote better health. It would seem that the maximum health benefits would be achieved by reducing our intake of meat and meat products, increasing our intake of complex carbohydrate, especially fiber, and decreasing our salt intake by relying less on processed foods and salting our own food much less. I am not suggesting becoming a vegetarian, although certainly this is an acceptable method of getting good nutrition, but I am encouraging our population to move more in that direction by replacing some of the large amounts of meat and dairy products we consume with complex carbohydrates, which contain fewer calories, less fat, and more fiber. Fortunately in the last few years there has been a trend toward this type of eating pattern. We as physicians should encourage that trend.

THE VEGETARIAN DIET

Vegetarianism, which is gaining more and more acceptance in western society, is the most widely practiced dietary pattern in many parts of the world. Therefore it cannot be considered a special diet, but rather an alternative to the usual eating patterns practiced in many countries. There are two major types of vegetarians, vegans, or those who consume foods of plant origin only, and ovolacto vegetarians, or those who consume foods of plant origin along with eggs and milk products. The latter diet is perfectly acceptable from every standpoint and will provide adequate amounts of all essential nutrients when properly practiced. The former, if strictly practiced, must be approached with some care and should be supplemented with at least one nutrient, vitamin B_{12}.

Ovolacto Vegetarian Diet

The limiting nutrients in any diet derived from plant origin are protein, iron, and vitamin B_{12}. If adequate amounts of animal products such as eggs, milk, and cheese, are consumed, then these nutrients will be provided in sufficient quantities to meet all requirements. Anyone who follows this diet must be warned of the danger of overconsumption of saturated fat and cholesterol as a result of eating large amounts of egg yolks, whole milk, and various cheeses. In addition, it should be noted that most cheeses contain large amounts of sodium and hence may have to be curtailed if sodium restriction is desired. This diet, however, is usually rich in protein and will contain adequate amounts of iron and vitamin B_{12}. The amount of calcium consumed is usually quite high, and the relatively low phosphorus favors calcium absorption. Thus the ovolacto vegetarian need not be strictly supervised unless serum cholesterol levels are such as to require dietary fat restriction. If they are, then simply reducing the number of egg yolks to two per week and changing from butter to a soft margarine will usually solve the problem. If the person is hypertensive and some sodium restriction is desired, then cheeses of most types should be discouraged and the use of natural rather than processed vegetables encouraged. Occasionally a person with lactose intolerance will choose to follow such a diet. Such people will usually seek their own safe levels of lactose intake and will voluntarily limit their intake of milk and certain cheeses. If they do not, the physician may have to recommend such limitations.

The Vegan Diet

This diet allows consumption of nutrients from plant origin only. Hence no meat or meat products, fish shellfish, eggs, and so on are consumed. With the exception of vitamin B_{12} and possibly iron, all of the required nutrients can be obtained in this diet. The most important consideration is meeting protein requirements. In general, plant proteins are incomplete. That is, they are missing one or more amino acids essential in human nutrition. By contrast, animal proteins, such as casein, egg albumin, or meat or fish proteins, will contain all of the essential amino acids. Therefore, to obtain an adequate amount of usable protein, an individual consuming a vegan diet either must eat liberal amounts of the relatively few vegetables that contain complete proteins, such as legumes, soya beans, and certain nuts, or must consume protein from several different vegetable sources which complement each other. This concept of complementing proteins has been empirically practiced by many civilizations for thousands of years. For example, Latin Americans consume corn (tortillas) and beans. Corn is relatively rich in trypophan but very poor in lysine. By contrast, beans contain lysine but little tryptophan. When consumed together, tortillas and beans *complement* each other and supply a complete source of protein. It is important to remember that complementary proteins must be eaten together for the individual to receive a complete protein. Table 1 is a listing of proteins from vegetable sources that complement each other. As one can see, with a little care it is relatively easy to supply adequate protein on a vegan diet. One particular concern should be noted in this regard. With the increased trend toward vegan families, we are seeing more and more small children weaned to diets of pure plant origin. The weanling child is particularly prone to protein deficiency (see Chapter 2) and cases of protein-calorie malnutrition and even of frank kwashiorkor are appearing with alarming frequency. It is very important at this stage of life to encourage the consumption of adequate amounts of *complete* protein. This means either continuing milk or milk products beyond the weaning period, supplying complete vegetable protein, or carefully complementing plant proteins in a way that the child will consume. To this end, peanut butter can and probably does serve a useful purpose. The same end can be achieved using soya beans or lentils. The growth and development of children growing up in a vegan family should be carefully monitored. This is the best way to ensure a diet adequate in protein.

Vitamin B_{12} is available only from animal sources. Hence a strict vegetarian will become deficient in vitamin B_{12}. Since symptoms of this deficiency often take a long time to develop, especially when the supply of folic acid is adequate, it is often overlooked. People consuming a vegan diet must be provided with a source of vitamin B_{12}. One source usually acceptable to the individual is brewer's yeast. A second is fortified breakfast cereal, and a third is direct vitamin supplementation.

Iron intake can also be a problem. The richest sources of iron are those foods in which the iron is present in the heme molecule, such as red meats and liver. Another good source is egg yolks. These sources are not available to the individual on a vegan diet. Vegetable sources provide inorganic iron and unless the diet is carefully chosen, deficiency can occur. Ingestion of high amounts of ascorbic acid, which often occurs on a vegan diet, will help by promoting iron absorption. However, all strict vegetarians must be considered at risk for iron deficiency. There are several ways to approach this problem. One is to explain to the patient that unless supple-

Table 1. Complementary proteins from plant sources

Plant Source	Amino Acids Missing from Protein	Complementary Protein Combinations
Grains	Isoleucine	Rice + legumes
	Lysine	Corn + legumes
		Wheat + legumes
		Wheat + peanut + milk
		Wheat + sesame + soybean
		Rice + brewer's yeast
Legumes	Tryptophan	Legumes + rice
	Methionine	Beans + wheat
		Beans + corn
		Soybeans + rice + wheat
		Soybeans + corn + milk
		Soybeans + wheat + sesame
		Soybeans + peanuts + sesame
		Soybeans + peanuts + wheat + rice
		Soybeans + sesame + wheat
Nuts and seeds	Isoleucine	Peanuts + sesame + soybeans
	Lysine	Sesame + beans
		Sesame + soybeans + wheat
		Peanuts + sunflower seeds
Vegetables	Isoleucine	Lima beans
	Methionine	Green beans
		Brussels sprouts } + sesame seeds or Brazil
		Cauliflower nuts or mushrooms
		Broccoli
		Greens + millet or rice

ments are consumed meal choices must be made bearing the iron content of the food in mind. Table 2 lists the iron content of certain vegetable foods that are relatively good sources of iron. A second approach is to encourage the consumption of iron-enriched foods, such as certain breakfast cereals. Finally, direct iron supplementation of 20 mg/day can be prescribed.

I believe iron supplementation is mandatory during certain periods of life in people consuming strictly vegetarian diets. These times include pregnancy, early childhood, and adolescence. In addition, any major loss of blood, even voluntary blood donation, should be treated by using supplementary iron.

Table 2.   Iron content of plant foods

Food	Amount (g)	Iron (mg)
Enriched white rice (cooked)	1 cup (205)	1.8
Brown rice (cooked)	1 cup (195)	1.0
Whole wheat bread (firm crumb)	1 slice (23)	0.7
Enriched white bread (firm crumb)	1 slice (23)	0.6
Whole egg (large, cooked)	1 (57)	1.2
Egg white (large)	1 (33)	0.02
Egg yolk (large, raw)	1 (17)	0.9
Spinach (leaf, frozen)	1 cup (190)	4.8
Kale (frozen)	1 cup (130)	1.3
Tofu	1 piece (120)	2.3
Peanuts	½ cup (72)	1.5
Raisins	1½ tbsp. (14)	0.5
Mung bean sprouts (raw)	1 cup (105)	1.4
Kidney beans (canned)	1 cup (255)	4.6
Lentil beans	1 cup (200)	4.2
Cheese (cheddar)	1 oz (28)	0.3
Brewer's yeast	1 tbsp. (8)	1.4
Torula yeast	1 oz. (28)	5.5
Peanut butter	2 tbsp. (32)	0.6
Banana (large)	1 (200)	1.0
Peach (large)	1 (175)	0.8
Apricots (dried, large)	5 halves (24)	1.3
Prunes (dried, large)	10 (97)	3.3
Potato (roasted in skin)	1 (202)	1.1

Calcium, though present in greatest amount in dairy products, is also present in certain foods of plant origin. Table 3 lists vegetarian foods that are rich in calcium. Since most people consuming a vegan diet will be ingesting relatively small amounts of phosphorus as well as protein, absorption of calcium will be very efficient and hence calcium supplementation is unnecessary. During pregnancy and lactation, however, when calcium requirements are very high, supplementation is recommended. This can be most easily accomplished by consuming 500 mg/day of calcium gluconate.

Thus the vegetarian, whether strict or including dairy products, can follow a healthful and varied diet with only minor adjustments. Such diets

Table 3. Plant sources of calcium

Food	Amount (g)	Calcium (mg)
Milk (all)	1 cup (244)	288
Yogurt (low fat)	1 cup (245)	294
Cheese (cheddar)	1 oz. (28)	213
Cottage cheese	$\frac{1}{2}$ cup (108)	100
Cheese (Swiss)	1 oz. (28)	260
Kale (frozen, cooked)	1 cup (130)	157
Almonds (whole)	1 cup (142)	332
Tofu	1 piece (120)	154
Molasses, blackstrap	2 tbsp. (40)	274
Tortillas	2	120

have the advantage of being high in fiber, and, in the case of strict vegetarians or those consuming only occasional dairy products, low in calories
and in total and saturated fat. A vegetarian diet is one way of consuming
the so-called prudent diet, and hence will offer a certain amount of protection against coronary disease. There is no reason for the physician to
discourage vegetarianism in anyone. Sometimes proper guidance is necessary. This is best achieved when we ourselves understand the strengths and
weaknesses of the particular type of vegetarian diet being consumed and
can explain the weaknesses and offer suggestions for correction to our
patients.

Macrobiotic Diets

These diets are forms of vegetarianism which become more and more
restrictive in the kinds of vegetables and fruits that can be consumed. In
their least restrictive form they may provide most essential nutrients and
may give the individual the opportunity to complement the kinds of proteins
that are permissible. In their most restrictive forms, when they allow only
herb teas and rice, they are deficient in most nutrients and if consumed for
any length of time can be dangerous. The forms between these extremes will
vary in their ability to provide one nutrient or another. In general, the
nutrients in the shortest supply are protein, iron, calcium, and vitamin
B_{12}. Children consuming certain macrobiotic diets and not exposed to
sunlight may develop rickets. The physician should determine as precisely
as possible what foods are actually being ingested and how much. From

the nature of the foods and their quantities, the nutrients most likely to be deficient can be deduced. With some understanding of the over-all dietary restriction imposed by the patient's particular regimen, certain simple and acceptable modifications are often possible. For example, the patient who is consuming only fruits and rice could benefit by the introduction of nuts, certain pulses, and other whole grains. Sometimes the diet is so rigid as to preclude any modifications within its structure that will ensure even moderately good nutrition. All the physician can do under these circumstances is to tell the patient what the potential problems are and to offer as many alternatives as possible for preventing these problems from occurring even if the alternatives fall outside the established rules for the particular diet being consumed.

Particular attention should be paid to pregnancy and lactation, since adherence to an extremely restrictive diet can affect fetal growth and development and deplete the nursing infant and mother. If this is carefully explained to the mother and careful modifications are worked out by mutual agreement, potentially dangerous problems can often be avoided. This kind of situation often takes considerable judgement, clinical skill, understanding, and above all the ability to work with the patient.

RECOMMENDED READING

Columbia University, Institute of Human Nutrition, *Nutrition and Health,* 1, No. 1-6 (1979).

Lappé, F. M., *Diet for a Small Planet,* 2nd ed., Ballantine, New York, 1975.

Select Committee on Nutrition and Human Needs, United States Senate, *Dietary Goals for the United States,* 2nd ed., United States Government Printing Office, Washington, D.C., 1977.

18

DISEASES OF THE GASTROINTESTINAL TRACT

Since the gastrointestinal (GI) tract is the normal route through which all nutrients must pass, diet plays a major role in the management of GI disease. Two types of disease processes within the GI tract have important nutritional implications:

1. Diseases in which contact with certain foods or particular nutrients will elicit symptoms, usually GI symptoms.
2. Diseases in which nutrients are improperly absorbed and consequently signs of nutrient deficiencies ensue.

In the first category are such diseases as peptic ulcer, gallbladder disease, hiatus hernia, chronic constipation, lactose intolerance, certain food allergies, and infant pyloric stenosis, and to some extent nonspecific diarrheas. Among those in the second category are the various diseases associated with malabsorption. Cystic fibrosis or other pancreatic disease, resection of large segments of the GI tract, and various infectious diarrheas, such as tropical sprue, are examples of this second category. Some of the most important gastrointestinal diseases show characteristics of both types of abnormality. Perhaps the best example is nontropical sprue, or celiac disease. The disease is caused by contact of a particular protein, gluten, with mucosal cells of the gastrointestinal tract. The response elicited by the GI tract is steatorrhea and severe malabsorption, which in turn often leads to severe nutrient deficiencies. Two other diseases, regional enteritis (Crohn's disease) and ulcerative colitis, can be viewed as showing characteristics of both categories. Ingestion of certain foods can aggravate the gastrointestinal symptoms and cause major discomfort to the patient. At the same time, both diseases, especially when severe enough, may result in malabsorption of certain nutrients.

USE OF DIET TO PREVENT OR ALLEVIATE SYMPTOMS

The most common disease in which diet has been used to alleviate symptoms is peptic ulcer. A mistake often made is the use of the so-called bland diets. These diets are often poorly defined and based on little or no experimental or clinical data. They are usually restrictive and may even result in iatrogenic nutrient deficiencies. At best, they sentence the patient, often for prolonged periods, to a dull, monotonous diet. At worst, they may be dangerous. Modern medical management of peptic ulcer should not include such a diet. The patient should be encouraged to eat whatever is not associated with pain or other symptoms. The major principle to follow is to keep the patient symptom free. Healing will usually follow as a natural consequence because the same factor, gastric acidity, is responsible for causing the symptoms and aggravating the lesion. Thus the best clinical evidence for healing is control of symptoms. In patients whose symptoms are controlled but whose lesion shows no radiographic signs of healing, malignancy must be suspected and surgery may be indicated.

There are, of course, certain principles that can be employed in the dietary management of patients with peptic ulcer. Anything that stimulates gastric acid secretion should be avoided. Coffee and alcohol are important in this respect. It is important to note that not only the caffeine in coffee but other ingredients as well stimulate excess acid secretion. Hence changing to decaffeinated coffee usually will not solve the problem. Coffee can be consumed occasionally and is much better tolerated after a meal, when the stomach is full, than between meals. This is also true of alcohol. Wine with the meal will cause much less trouble than one or two martinis before the meal. Antacids and buffering foods are useful in relief of pain. However, the patient should be warned against the overuse of milk and especially cream, which is very high in saturated fat and in calories, and which has resulted in the past in many ulcer patients' developing obesity and coronary artery disease. Although there is no doubt that the protein in cow's milk preparations will buffer acid, the relief is often short lived and there is some evidence that acid secretion may be stimulated by the protein content.

Today the patient with a peptic ulcer who is managed medically can be maintained on a relatively normal diet. The use of bland foods should be discouraged, and with the warnings described above, patients should be allowed to seek their own levels of tolerance to certain foods. The physician should offer alternatives if the diet is in anyway inadequate. Since at present we do not know any dietary factor or combination of factors that will directly promote healing, the best approach is to control the often severe symptoms. Fortunately, in most cases healing will follow this course of action. If healing does not occur, surgical treatment must be considered.

DIET IN PATIENTS WHO HAVE HAD GASTRIC SURGERY

There is always some derangement of GI function after gastric surgery. Weight loss is invariable after total gastrectomy and occurs quite often after partial gastrectomy. This is undoubtably because of the small capacity of the "stomach" in such patients and consequently the rapid feeling of fullness. In addition, a troublesome group of symptoms, referred to as the "dumping syndrome," occurs in a significant number of patients following partial gastrectomy. This syndrome is characterized by nausea, abdominal bloating, cramping pains, and diarrhea, as well as by certain vasomotor symptoms, such as sweating, palpitations, weakness, drowsiness, and dizziness, which occur within 5 minutes to $1\frac{1}{2}$ hours after eating. Therapy is not entirely satisfactory; however, some patients may lessen the symptoms by decreasing the quantity of food consumed at a single sitting or by avoiding certain foods which by experience they have discovered worsen the symptoms.

A small number of patients will develop reactive hypoglycemia following gastrectomy. These patients should be encouraged to consume liquids separately from (preferably before) solid foods. In addition, dry foods are preferred in frequent small meals. Finally, rapidly absorbed carbohydrates, such as simple sugars, should be avoided.

Another late complication of gastric surgery in a small number of patients is malabsorption and steatorrhea. The exact reason for this is not known, but it has been postulated to be caused by poor coordination between gastric emptying and gallbladder and pancreatic secretion. In some cases, bacterial overgrowth into the small intestines may occur. Treatment consists of antibiotics to control bacterial overgrowth, and the administration of pancreatic enzymes. In addition, if the steatorrhea is severe, medium-chain triglycerides should replace other sources of fat. Finally, a significant number of patients with partial gastrectomy and an even larger number following total gastrectomy will develop iron or vitamin

B_{12} deficiency. Iron should be supplemented orally and B_{12} levels monitored. If these levels are low, then B_{12} should be administered intramuscularly.

CHOLECYSTITIS

Acute or chronic inflammation of the gallbladder is most often due to an infection superimposed on a totally or partially obstructed gallbladder, usually by stones. During an acute attack the patient may be unable to take anything by mouth initially. Under these conditions, it is important to maintain adequate hydration and electrolyte balance, and intravenous fluids should be used. When foods by mouth can be introduced, fat should be avoided since stimulation of gallbladder contraction may exacerbate symptoms. Once the acute episode subsides if surgical therapy is not indicated a regular diet can be resumed. In chronic cholecystitis, if for any reason surgery is contraindicated, the patient will establish a dietary pattern that minimizes symptoms. Often this will involve curtailment of fried foods. Some fat should be included in the diet to ensure drainage of the gallbladder. Therapy in a sense is like that for peptic ulcer. No dietary regimen will cure the lesion; hence control of symptoms is the objective. In this the patient is often the best guide to successful therapy.

INTOLERANCE OF LACTOSE AND OTHER DISACCHARIDES

The management of lactose intolerance is discussed in Chapter 14. Occasionally, patients who are intolerant to other disaccharides are seen. The symptoms involve flatulence, abdominal pain, diarrhea, and acid stools. The diagnosis can be made by doing a loading test with the appropriate sugar (see Chapter 14), and if intolerance is demonstrated exclusion or marked reduction in the quantity of the offending sugar can be recommended.

PYLORIC STENOSIS

This disease, which is due to a congenital malformation of the pyloric musculature, manifests itself usually around the third week of life. Dietary management is mentioned only to be discouraged since surgical correction is simple and permanent. If for some reason surgery must be delayed, then thickened feedings (formula thickened with cereal) may be tolerated and parenteral nutrition avoided.

CHRONIC NONSPECIFIC DIARRHEA OF INFANCY

The principle of dietary management in this situation is to supply adequate nutrition to the patient without worsening the diarrhea and hence the nutrient loss. In the past this was often difficult since "resting the bowel" meant partially starving the patient. Thus feeding regimens were employed which were minimally irritating and supplied adequate amounts of nutrients. For relatively short lived diarrhea this approach may still be valid. However, for prolonged chronic diarrhea a period of total parenteral nutrition with nothing by mouth is indicated. Oral feedings can then be tried in very small amounts and slowly titrated to the patient's tolerance.

DISEASES ASSOCIATED WITH MALABSORPTION

Deficiency in Pancreatic Enzymes

The two diseases most often associated with pancreatic enzyme deficiency are cystic fibrosis and chronic pancreatitis.

Cystic Fibrosis

Cystic fibrosis is a genetically transmitted (autosomal recessive) disease involving the exocrine glands of the body. Secretion of abnormally viscous mucus leads to problems within the pulmonary system which are usually progressive and ultimately lead to the patient's death. Abnormal loss of sodium, potassium, and chloride through the sweat glands may lead to electrolyte derangements, especially in hot weather. In 80 to 90% of cases exocrine pancreatic insufficiency occurs as a result of obstruction of the ductiles and atrophy and fibrosis of the pancreatic exocrine tissue. The volume of pancreatic secretion is reduced. The pH becomes less alkaline and the quantity of all of the pancreatic enzymes is greatly reduced. As a consequence of these changes, malabsorption of protein, fat, complex carbohydrates, vitamins, and certain minerals will result.

Treatment consists of adequate oral supplementation with pancreatic enzymes, a high carbohydrate, low fat diet, supplementation of all vitamins (parenterally if necessary), and added sodium chloride as well as calcium and magnesium. If adequate caloric intake cannot be maintained, medium-chain triglycerides can be used as a source of calories since these do not require pancreatic lipase or bile salts for their absorption. Finally, amino acid supplements given with meals may be necessary in certain cases, particularly if an adequate growth rate is not maintained.

As a consequence of better pulmonary management more and more patients with cystic fibrosis are reaching adulthood. As a result, a long-term complication is being seen with increased frequency: focal biliary cirrhosis secondary to intrahepatic cholangiolar plugging. This may lead to portal hypertension and all of its attendant complications.

Chronic Pancreatitis

Although this disease may have a variety of causes, in the United States alcoholism is by far the most common. The functional abnormality is similar to that observed with cystic fibrosis. However, the pancreatic insufficiency is rarely as severe and since it occurs in adults the nutritional requirements are not as great. Most patients can therefore be managed by oral supplementation with pancreatic enzyme alone. In those who cannot tolerate enzyme therapy well or who are not controlled by enzymes alone, medium-chain triglycerides and amino acid mixtures may be used. The patient's weight should be carefully monitored to assess adequacy of therapy.

Blind Loop Syndromes

This syndrome occurs when for any one of a number of reasons associated with degenerative or inflammatory disease of the bowel or surgical procedures there is bacterial overgrowth into the small intestine. Dilations proximal to strictures, diverticuli, and surgical constructions of cul-de-sacs which do not drain adequately supply sites where bacteria can flourish and multiply rapidly. The major nutrients that are poorly absorbed are fat and vitamin B_{12}. The steatorrhea may secondarily impair absorption of fat-soluble vitamins and of certain minerals, such as calcium and magnesium. The steatorrhea is believed to be induced by bacterial deconjugation of bile salts, which renders them unable to assist in the formation of micelles. The B_{12} malabsorption appears to be caused by sequestration of vitamin B_{12} by the bacteria.

If surgical correction is possible to relieve the area of stasis and improve drainage, this is the treatment of choice. When it is not possible, antibiotic treatment may control the bacterial overgrowth, although only rarely can the bacteria be entirely eradicated in this manner. Therefore, some symptoms will remain and dietary management is important. This includes the use of medium-chain triglycerides by mouth and vitamin B_{12} parenterally.

Tropical Sprue

This disease, endemic in certain areas of the tropics, especially Southeast Asia, is characterized by sore mouth, steatorrhea, and secondary general malnutrition. The malabsorption that occurs in this disease, while primarily involving fat, includes water, electrolytes, glucose, vitamins, and minerals. The etiology is unknown. Pathological changes are nonspecific, involving atrophy of the jejunal villi similar to the atrophy seen in gluten enteropathy.

Dietary therapy involves high protein, low fat, and low carbohydrate foods (medium-chain triglycerides may be used). Vitamin and mineral supplementation is essential, particularly with folic acid (especially if glossitis, stomatitis, or macrocytosis is present) and vitamin K (especially if a hemorrhagic diathesis is present).

Short Bowel Syndrome

Up to 40% of the small intestine can be resected without causing major problems as long as the duodenum, distal ileum, and ileocecal valve are left intact. More extensive resection or removal of a significant amount of distal ileum or the ileocecal valve may result in significant malabsorption, the severity of which will depend on the extent of resection, the site of resection, and the presence of remaining diseased segments. The major reason for having to undertake extensive bowel resection is ischemia due to thrombosis or embolism. Other reasons are Crohn's disease, trauma, and malignancy. Malabsorption of all nutrients may take place. Initially fluid loss following surgery is extensive, requiring parenteral nutrition. In some cases, this will persist and any oral feedings will aggravate the diarrhea and fluid loss. In the past, such patients died of progressive malnutrition. At present, long-term parenteral nutrition carried out at home is maintaining a number of such patients in satisfactory nutritional condition and allowing them to live a reasonably normal life (see Chapter 22). Most patients, however, can be controlled with careful dietary management. This includes frequent high protein meals with carbohydrate and fat to the patient's level of tolerance. Medium-chain triglycerides may be given to increase calories. Vitamins should be given by mouth and if terminal ileum has been resected, 100 mg of vitamin B_{12} must be given by injection every 3 to 4 weeks. Calcium and magnesium supplementation may be necessary, as well as anticholinergic drugs to reduce diarrhea.

Radiation Enteritis

The commonest disease of the small bowel resulting in a malabsorption syndrome is radiation disease secondary to radiotherapy for pelvic or retroperitoneal malignancy. Mucosal cell turnover is inhibited, epithelial integrity is breached, and secondary bacterial infection may occur. The subacute and more chronic effects cause vascular changes such as obliterative endarteritis, which is followed by fibrosis and stricture. A generalized malabsorption syndrome will occur which is similar to that seen in regional enteritis (Crohn's disease) and the treatment is therefore the same.

Regional Enteritis (Crohn's Disease)

Nonspecific regional enteritis (Crohn's disease) is a disease of unknown etiology in which there is inflammation of the small bowel usually involving the terminal ileum. Mucosal damage leading to fibrosis and stricture formation occurs in more severe cases. Symptoms include cramping pains and diarrhea, and in more serious cases various degrees of malabsorption.

Since the terminal 90 cm of the ileum is where vitamin B_{12} and bile salts are absorbed for enterohepatic recirculation, malabsorption of this vitamin and of fat will occur in regional enteritis if the disease is severe enough. The unabsorbed bile salts may further irritate the bowel, causing diarrhea. If the involvement of small intestine is more widespread, not only fat but protein and even carbohydrate may be malabsorbed.

Treatment involves the use of a high carbohydrate, high protein, low fat diet. If protein malabsorption is present, amino acids can replace some or most of the protein. Medium-chain triglycerides can be used to replace some of the fat, and if necessary an exchange resin, cholestyramine, may be given to remove irritating bile salts. Since committing the patient to long-term intramuscular injections with vitamin B_{12} is unconfortable and expensive, preliminary absorption tests should be carried out to determine if absorption is defective. Since the disease may have a tendency to improve and relapse spontaneously, it is often necessary to use parenteral nutrition temporarily to tide the patient over a particularly serious episode. Some patients after prolonged disease and multiple surgical procedures need long-term parenteral nutrition, but this number fortunately is quite small.

Gluten Enteropathy (Nontropical Sprue, Celiac Disease)

This disease occurs in both a juvenile and an adult form. In children it usually presents during the first 3 years of life with failure to thrive, loss of appetite, and a characteristic pot-bellied appearance, as shown in Figure 1.

Stunting of growth and infantile development will occur if the disease remains untreated for a long time. Large, bulky, pale, foul smelling stools are due to the malabsorption and the presence of free fatty acids.

The clinical features of the adult onset disease are indistinguishable from those of tropical sprue, including the mouth lesions and the malabsorption. In both adults and children the disease is caused by an idiosyncrasy or sensitivity to gluten, which is a mixture of proteins found in certain grains (primarily wheat and rye). The actual offending substance is gliadin. There is evidence that a particular fraction of gliadin damages the intestinal mucosa and it has been suggested that an enzyme or enzymes

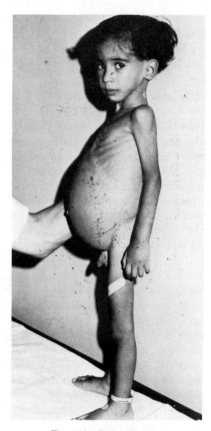

Figure 1. Celiac disease.

necessary for the digestion of this fraction are missing in patients with this disease. Whatever the mechanism involved, the treatment is the same—exclusion of gluten from the diet. This is a difficult task and requires the cooperation of the patient and careful management by a skilled dietician. Table 1 lists some common foods containing gluten, such as wheats, oats, rye, barley, and buckwheat, which must be omitted from the diet, and some foods that are gluten free, which may be used. If a particular food is in doubt there are lists that can be consulted. If in doubt it is better to omit the food, since even small amounts of gluten can precipitate an attack.

In children who have suffered from the disease for a short time response to a gluten free diet is often rapid (within a few weeks). In patients who have suffered for a prolonged period, particularly adults, the response may take much longer (3 to 6 months for complete recovery). Anemia is often present in both children and adults. In children it is most often microcytic hypochromic anemia due to iron deficiency; in adults it is usually megaloblastic anemia due to folic acid deficiency. Until the symp-

Table 1. Gluten content of some common foods [a]

Present (foods that must be avoided)	Bread, biscuits, cakes, cookies, crackers, doughnuts, flour (white or wholewheat), muffins, pancakes, pastry, pies, pretzels, rolls, waffles, breakfast cereals made with wheat or oatmeal. Pasta, any meat containing filler, i.e., commercial hamburger or hotdogs, canned meat, meatloaf, canned soups or soup mixes, vegetables with cream sauces or crumbs, sauces, ketchup, gravies or salad dressings commercially available, malted milk, beer, commercial milk flavorings, baking powder, cheese spreads, most ice creams, commercial chocolates
Absent (foods that may be eaten)	Milk (all kinds), yogurt, fresh meat or poultry, bacon, fish (fresh or canned), shellfish, organ meats, gravies made with cornstarch or rice flour. Cheese, egg in any form, vegetables (fresh, frozen, canned), potatoes, rice, nuts, all fruits and fruit juices, bread and flour made from arrowroot, cornmeal, potato, soybean, or rice flour, breakfast cereals made from rice or corn (Rice Krispies or cornflakes), fats and oils, butter, margarine, peanut butter, sugar, jam, jelly, marmalade, honey, syrup, hard candies, homemade chocolate, desserts made with gelatin, tapioca, sage, rice and cornstarch, coffee, tea, carbonated beverages, salt, pepper, mustard, garlic, spices, vinegar

[a] Adapted from Davidson, 1975.

toms have disappeared on a gluten free diet, specific replacement with iron or folic acid should be carried out.

Although some children may have to remain on a gluten free diet for the rest of their lives, others develop a tolerance for gluten. Hence, after at least 5 years of satisfactory dietary control, an attempt can be made to introduce foods containing gluten. If symptoms occur, immediate return to the diet is indicated. Even if there are no overt symptoms, periodic checks for anemia and steatorrhea should be made. In adults, complete recovery is much less likely and dietary management is usually permanent.

Ulcerative Colitis

This disease is the most frequent cause of chronic diarrhea in adults in temperate climates. It is characterized by blood and mucus in the stool secondary to an inflammatory reaction in the large intestine which is manifested by mucosal ulceration. No pathogenic organism has been identified with the disease. There is an association between ulcerative colitis and certain autoimmune diseases. In most cases there are serious psychological disturbances, but whether these are cause or effect is not clear. In a small number of cases an intestinal allergy may be the cause of the disease, and such patients may respond to withdrawal of milk or milk products. Some cases of unrecognized lactose intolerance may simulate ulcerative colitis after a long time.

The disease is usually cyclic, with the patient suffering from acute attacks followed by periods of relative quiescence.

Dietary management is extremely important, especially when the patient is having an acute episode. Fluids, electrolytes, and blood may have to be replaced intravenously. Oral treatment should include a high protein diet built around egg, meat, and vegetable proteins, and milk proteins if they are tolerated. Carbohydrate content of the diet should be high, and if fat is tolerated it is permissible. If not, medium-chain triglycerides in a palatable form may be tried. Vitamins should be supplemented. Citrus fruits and other laxative foods should be omitted during an attack and taken with caution and moderation between attacks. Although dietary treatment is extremely important, other modes of therapy are often indicated. These include the use of corticosteroids, sulfa drugs, and psychotherapy. Under extreme conditions surgical resection is called for.

RECOMMENDED READING

Ament, M. E., Malabsorption Syndromes in Infancy and Childhood, *J. Pediat.*, **81,** 685; 867 (1972).

Crane, R. K., A Perspective of Digestion-Absorptive Function, *Am. J. Clin. Nutr.*, **22**, 242 (1969).

Davidson, S., R. Passmore, J. F. Brock, and A. S. Truswell, *Human Nutrition and Dietetics*, Churchill Livingstone, Edinburgh, 1975, Chapter 41.

Danielsson, H., Influence of Bile Acids on Digestion and Absorption of Lipids, *Am. J. Clin. Nutr.*, **12**, 214 (1963).

Gray, G. M., Drugs, Malnutrition, and Carbohydrate Absorption, *Am. J. Clin. Nutr.*, **26**, 121 (1973).

Haenel, H., Human Normal and Abnormal Gastrointestinal Flora, *Am. J. Clin. Nutr.*, **26**, 121 (1973).

Ingelfinger, F. J., Gastrointestinal Absorption, *Nutr. Today*, **2**, 2 (1967).

Isselbacher, K. J., Metabolism and Transport of Lipids by Intestinal Mucosa, *Fed. Proc.*, **24**, 16 (1965).

Rosensweig, N. S., R. H. Herman, and F. B. Stifel, Dietary Regulation of Small Intestine Enzyme Activity in Man, *Am. J. Clin. Nutr.*, **24**, 65 (1971).

Spencer, R. P., Intestinal Absorption of Amino Acids, Current Concepts, *Am. J. Clin. Nutr.*, **22**, 292 (1969).

Symposium on Mechanisms of Gastrointestinal Absorption, *Am. J. Clin. Nutr.*, **12**, 161 (1963).

Taylor, K. B., Gastroenterology, in H. A. Schneider, C. E. Anderson, and D. B. Coursin, Eds., *Nutritional Support of Medical Practice*, Harper and Row, Hagerstown, Md., 1977, pp. 332–340.

Underwood, B. A., and C. R. Denning, Blood and Liver Concentrations of Vitamin A and E in Children with Cystic Fibrosis of the Pancreas, *Pediat. Res.*, **6**, 26 (1972).

Winick, M., Ed., *Nutrition and Gastroenterology*, Wiley, New York, 1980.

19

HYPERTENSION

Cardiovascular disease is the leading cause of death among people living in developed countries. Coronary artery disease and cerebrovascular accidents account for the greatest number of these deaths. As we have seen, both of these diseases are multifactorial in origin and are more common in individuals manifesting certain risk factors. The most important of these risk factors are cigarette smoking, hyperlipidemia, hypertension, and diabetes. In addition, obesity, by contributing to the last three, is an important indirect risk factor in cardiovascular disease. Except for cigarette smoking, all the major risk factors are related to nutrition. The level of serum lipids can be influenced by the amount of saturated fat and cholesterol in the diet and hence a prudent diet as discussed in Chapter 3 is indicated in any individual who manifests evidence of hyperlipidemia or who has a family history of cardiovascular disease. In fact, a movement in the direction of the prudent diet would be beneficial to the public in general. The major benefit of this diet is preventing progression of the disease. Although there is some evidence that some reversal of the disease process itself can occur, the results in this regard are not dramatic. Hence although anyone who has had a heart attack should be maintained on a diet low in saturated fat and cholesterol, in a strict sense, this diet cannot be considered a therapeutic diet.

By contrast, hypertension can be at least partially controlled, after it occurs, by dietary means. Hypertension, defined as a blood pressure consistently higher than 140 systolic and 90 diastolic, is probably the most significant risk factor for cardiovascular disease. It is related to atherosclerosis, cerebrovascular accidents, congestive heart failure, renal failure, coronary occlusion, and angina pectoris. Hypertension increases the severity of a heart attack when it occurs. About 50% of hypertensives have enlarged hearts and many develop kidney disease and eventual kidney failure. Hypertension is a silent disease, often manifesting no symptoms before a catastrophic complication ensues. Thus not only must a careful blood pressure determination be part of every physical examination, but mass screening programs should be encouraged and people advised to have their blood pressure determined semiannually. This is extremely important because hypertension often strikes in the so-called healthy years when patients may visit a physician infrequently. Results of such screening procedures have revealed that about 20% of white adult males and nearly 50% of black adult males are hypertensives.

Hypertension may be the result of definable organic pathology and therefore its causes deserve investigation. In a small number of cases renal disease will be uncovered. In an even smaller number rare conditions such as pheochromocytoma or adrenal tumors may produce hypertension. In most cases, however, no direct cause for the hypertension will be uncovered. This so-called idiopathic hypertension can be divided into two major types: malignant hypertension and essential hypertension. The former is relatively rare and will progress rapidly to death if untreated. The disease occurs more frequently in younger individuals and is characterized by extreme elevations of blood pressure, blurring of vision, headache, dyspnea, and renal failure. Treatment consists of management with one or more antihypertensive agents. The more common type is essential hypertension. Usually an elevated blood pressure is the only sign of the disease. There does not appear to be any single cause of essential hypertension. Both animal experiments and studies in human populations strongly implicate a genetic predisposition. In addition, certain environmental conditions, especially in genetically susceptible populations, are important. Nutrition plays a central role among the environmental conditions that predispose to hypertension. Obesity and excess intake of sodium have both been implicated in the etiology of the disease, and patients with essential hypertension will often respond to weight reduction and sodium removal. Weight reduction in a patient with essential hypertension is no different from weight reduction in any obese patient, and dietary management should be approached as discussed in Chapter 12. Crash diets, especially those based on extremely high protein intake, should be discouraged. The patient must learn that a potentially serious complication of obesity has occurred and that a mainstay of treatment is losing weight *and keeping it off.* Even patients who are only moderately overweight should be encouraged to lose weight. Often weight reduction alone will result in a return of the blood pressure to normal. Even if total normality is not achieved significant lowering of the blood pressure can be expected in most cases.

Reducing the amount of sodium retained by the body by limiting sodium intake is a much more difficult task even than weight control, because to achieve a low enough sodium intake needed if sodium restriction alone is to be employed a major change in lifestyle is required.

As has been discussed in Chapter 15, the normal adult requires approximately 0.5 g/day of sodium. The average level of consumption in the United States is 6 to 8 g/day. Most patients with essential hypertension will not respond unless intake is reduced to levels near the actual requirement. This, for many people, is an extremely restrictive diet. Hence, for most people with hypertension, mild or moderate salt restriction coupled with the use of diuretic agents (which promote sodium excretion) is the treatment of choice. The major exception is the patient with congestive heart failure, who should be maintained on very strict salt restriction as well as diuretics and digitalis.

From a practical standpoint, then, sodium-restricted diets can be divided into three main categories:

1. Mild or 2 g/day.
2. Moderate or 1 g/day
3. Strict or 0.5 g/day.

For mild restriction, one simply reduces the amount of table salt used. No salt should be added at the table, but up to 1 teaspoon per day can be added during cooking. In addition, pickled foods (sauerkraut, pickled fish, sour pickles, and smoked fish) and extremely salty foods (luncheon meats, snack chips, and processed cheeses) should be eliminated. Table 1 lists foods that should be eliminated from the diet because of their high sodium content.

For most individuals suffering from essential hypertension with moderate elevations of blood pressure (140 to 180 systolic and 90 to 100 diastolic) this type of diet, along with a diuretic which promotes sodium excretion, will bring blood pressure into the normal range, especially if some weight reduction has been accomplished.

The moderately restricted diet prohibits the use of salt at the table but allows the use of 1/4 teaspoon per day in cooking. This diet limits the form of a food eaten rather than imposing any limitations on the actual foods consumed beyond those outlined on the mildly restricted diet. Corn, for example, is permitted if eaten fresh, frozen unsalted, or canned unsalted. The same is true for all other vegetables, fruits, meats, fish, poultry, fats, and grains. The person should consume unsalted or low sodium dairy products, breads, and cereals. However, to allow flexibility in the diet, up to three servings a day are permitted from restricted foods. This means

Table 1.   Foods to omit on a sodium-restricted diet

Food	Level of Restriction		
	Mild	Moderate	Strict
Fruits	All forms are permitted (including fresh, frozen, canned, and dried)		
Vegetables, soups, and vegetable juices	Omit pickled and dehydrated forms		
	No additional restrictions	Limit canned to 2 servings daily	Omit all canned and frozen if processed with salt. Omit all in Table 2
Meats Fish Poultry Eggs	Omit cold cuts, sausages, cured and pickled products		
	No additional restrictions	Limit canned to 2 servings daily	Omit all canned or frozen with salt
Bread and grain products	Omit salted crackers, pretzels, etc.		
	No additional restrictions	Limit ready-to-eat and "quick cooking" cereals, commercial bread, or baked products to 3 servings daily	Omit all products prepared with sodium
Milk and dairy products	Omit all cheeses and cheese spreads		
	No additional restrictions	Limit fluid milk and milk products to 3 servings daily	Omit all but low sodium products
Seasonings	Omit boullion, dehydrated soup, and soy sauce		
	Limit salt to 1 tsp.	Limit salt to 1/4 tsp.	Omit all salt, salted butter or margarine
	No additional restrictions	Omit catsup, mustard, commercial salad preparations, and seasoning salts	

that a salad bar which offers an array of fresh vegetables along with several dishes of canned beets or canned chickpeas can be fully utilized. Table 1 outlines the options on a moderate restriction more fully.

Moderate restriction of salt intake combined with weight reduction and a diuretic agent will bring most cases of even severe essential hypertension under control. For those individuals whose hypertension cannot be controlled using this approach or who are suffering from congestive heart failure due to myocardial damage no matter what the etiology, strict sodium restriction is indicated. This diet permits no salt at the table, no salt added in cooking, no foods processed with salt (see Table 1) and no foods naturally high in sodium (Table 2). Thus the diet is restricted to foods naturally low in sodium (Table 3).

Table 2.   Vegetables naturally high in sodium

Artichokes	Celery flakes	Whole hominy	Parsely flakes
Beet greens	Chard	Kale	Spinach
Carrots	Dandelion greens	Mustard Greens	White turnip
Celery			

Table 3.   Foods with insignificant amounts of sodium—permitted for all diets

Grains	Wheat, oats, rye, rice, barley, and their products (e.g., pasta, breads, flours, uncooked cereals)
Vegetables	All those not in Table 2 or canned/frozen salt-free
Fruits	All fresh/canned fruits and all juices
Meats	All fresh or frozen/canned without salt beef, lamb, pork, veal, poultry, fish, shellfish, and game meats
Eggs	All fresh
Fats	All vegetable oils and shortenings, lard, and unsalted butter and margarine
Condiments	Vinegar, all spices, mustard powder, flavorings that do not contain salt
Sweeteners	Sugar, honey, syrup, jellies, molasses
Beverages	Alcoholic beverages, coffee, teas, soft drinks

As can be seen, this diet is more difficult to follow than the other two especially for meals consumed out of the home. In our society, it virtually precludes eating in fast food chains and markedly reduces the options even in the best restaurants. For this reason, it is used only if no other alternative is available.

RECOMMENDED READING

Columbia University Institute of Human Nutrition, *Nutrition and Health,* **1**, No. 3 (Hypertension) (1979).

Committee on Nutrition, American Academy of Pediatrics, Salt Intake and Eating Patterns of Infants and Children in Relation to Blood Pressure, *Pediatrics,* **53**, 115 (1974).

Dahl, L. K., Salt and Hypertension, *Am. J. Clin. Nutr.,* **25**, 231 (1972).

Meneely, G. R., and H. D. Battarbee, Sodium and Potassium, in *Present Knowledge in Nutrition,* The Nutrition Foundation, Washington, D.C., 1976, pp. 259–279.

Tobian, L., Jr., Hypertension and the Kidney, *Arch. Int. Med.,* **133**, 959 (1974).

20

RENAL DISEASE

Since the kidney is the major excretory organ for the end products of metabolic processes involved in the utilization of many exogenous nutrients, the nutritional management of the patient with renal disease is a crucial factor in reducing mortality and morbidity.

The most common renal problems necessitating careful dietary management are chronic renal failure (from whatever cause), acute renal failure (usually due to trauma, burns, or surgery), and the nephrotic syndrome. Each of these conditions requires nutritional management whose strategy is quite different and is based on the pathophysiologic changes attendant on the particular disease.

CHRONIC RENAL FAILURE

The common denominator in all patients with chronic renal failure is the inability to excrete nitrogen properly. As a result, the levels of nonprotein nitrogen products increase in the blood. As the levels of these products increase, particularly urea, the patient begins to develop certain symptoms and is said to be suffering from uremia. The major aims of therapy under these conditions are to prevent further strain on the system by limiting the amount of exogenous nitrogen ingested and to create conditions whereby the body is able to convert the excess nonprotein nitrogen (urea and ammonia) into utilizable amino acids. In addition, it is important to create conditions that minimize breakdown of endogenous proteins (from muscle and other sources).

The first aim is best accomplished by limiting the amount of protein in the diet. This was realized 50 years ago when low protein diets were introduced in the treatment of uremic patients. Unfortunately, such diets had only limited success because the protein supplied was derived from the usual sources (simply in reduced amounts) rather than limited to protein of high biologic value. After the concept of essential amino acids was clearly understood, it became clear that the liver could synthesize all of the other, nonessential, amino acids from carbohydrate and nonprotein nitrogen sources. Hence, not only did protein have to be restricted but the requirement for all of the essential amino acids had to be met at the same time in order for the endogenous urea to be converted to nonessential amino acids and utilized in normal body protein turnover.

In 1963, Giordano introduced this concept into the feeding of patients with chronic renal disease. By feeding 2 g/day of essential amino acid nitrogen as the sole source of nitrogen and by ensuring adequate calories, vitamins, and minerals, he was able to induce a decline in blood urea nitrogen (BUN) and a reduction of endogenous protein catabolism. The nitrogen balance of the patients became positive and many of their uremic symptoms disappeared. These studies demonstrated that endogenous urea could be utilized in the synthesis of nonessential amino acids but that for such utilization to occur essential amino acids and calories had to be supplied in adequate amounts. In addition, exogenous nonessential amino acids had to be restricted to encourage the utilization of urea. These carefully conducted clinical studies implied that the optimum diet for patients with uremia was a diet limited in protein and restricted to protein of high biologic value (high essential amino acid content) coupled with sufficient calories (from nonprotein sources) for normal metabolism.

In 1964, Giovannetti and Maggiore utilized these implications in the direct management of patients with chronic renal failure. They fed these patients a high calorie, low protein diet and either powdered essential amino acids or eggs. The egg protein was able to substitute for the essential amino acid mixture because of its very high biologic value which ensured adequate supplies of the eight essential amino acids and minimal amounts of nonessential amino acids. Initially, the patients were given wafers prepared from maize starch and spaghetti from low protein wheat to supply adequate calories and minimal nonessential amino acids. At first, these patients were in negative nitrogen balance but their BUN declined and their uremic symptoms improved. After 5 to 10 days, the powdered essential amino acids (1.74 g of nitrogen) or the egg albumin (1.5 to 2.2 g of nitrogen) was added. Nitrogen balance became positive, BUN continued to drop, and symptoms improved further.

This so-called Giovanetti diet has been modified several times in different countries to appeal more to the tastes of the local populations. In Britain, for example, an 18 to 21 g protein diet was fed from the onset with 12 g supplied as egg or milk. Except for methionine, this diet supplied the minimum daily requirement of all essential amino acids. Therefore, a supplement of 500 mg of methionine was given. Bread and other special products were developed which were low in protein and were utilized to minimize ingestion of nonessential amino acids and to increase caloric intake.

Whether protein intake should be controlled depends on the degree of renal functional impairment and on the signs and symptoms displayed by the patient. Table 1 outlines the current guidelines employed by the group at the Mayo Clinic and the amount of protein permitted under various conditions. Renal function is determined by creatinine clearance.

Protein restriction is instituted only when creatinine clearance has dropped below 30 ml/min/1.73 m^2. These recommendations may have to be adjusted in any individual case since some patients may require more or less protein restriction. The source of the protein must be of high biologic value, preferably egg or milk. If protein is being lost in the urine, the amount lost should be determined and replaced in the diet over and above the recommendations in Table 1.

If the patient's symptoms preclude the ingestion of the diet, peritoneal dialysis may be necessary to obtain inital relief. If renal symptoms are such that repeated hemodialysis is necessary, the above management should be used until the dialysis program is instituted and then the protein intake should be increased to 0.75 to 1.0 g/kg. If successful renal transplant is accomplished, no further protein restriction is necessary.

Generous caloric intake should be maintained to minimize muscle catabolism. Nonobese patients should consume 1800 to 3500 kcal/day, depending on height, weight, age, sex, and activity. This level can be achieved by supplying large amounts of carbohydrates, which are best consumed along with the protein or within 4 hours of protein ingestion. Low protein wheat starch products are used as the primary source of high

Table 1. Protein intake according to the degree of renal failure

Creatinine Clearance (ml/min/1.73 m^2)	Daily Protein Intake	
	g/kg Body Weight	g/70 kg Man
30–20	0.7–0.5	49–35
19–5	0.38	27
5	0.26	18

calorie food. Several such products are on the market and can be used in preparing bread, cakes, puddings, and pancakes. A 40 g slice of wheat starch bread supplies approximately 0.2 g of protein and 115 kcal. By contrast, the usual 25 g slice of regular bread supplies ten times the protein and just over half the calories. In addition, there are a number of high calorie carbohydrate powders which are protein free and can be consumed either with water or with juice or can be added in cooking. While some caloric reduction may be useful in obese patients with mild renal failure, restriction of calories in patients with severe disease (creatinine clearance less than 15 ml/min/1.73 m^2) is not advised because of the danger of increasing muscle catabolism and thereby elevating the BUN.

Some patients with chronic renal failure will tend to retain sodium and may develop hypertension and edema. Others will lose sodium and may become dehydrated. A 24 hour urinary sodium determination is invaluable in determining the patient's sodium status. If sodium is being retained, a low sodium diet should be instituted, with the degree of restriction slowly increased until urinary sodium excretion approaches intake. By contrast, if sodium is being lost in the urine, salt can be added to foods to bring intake and output into equilibrium. In patients with severe hypertension and edema, strict sodium restriction (to less than 500 mg/day) may have to be instituted. This should be done only as a last resort, since the diet is extremely restrictive and imposes added burdens on a patient whose diet is already restrictive. For this reason antihypertensive drugs should be employed to control the hypertension, and salt restriction combined with such therapy should be used only to the extent necessary.

Vitamins and other minerals may be depleted in patients with chronic renal disease, especially if they are consuming the type of diet outlined above. Therefore, a multivitamin capsule along with 5 mg of extra folic acid and 1 to 3 g of calcium given as calcium carbonate are recommended. If the patient is hypercalcemic, the calcium supplement should be omitted. If the product of calcium and phosphorus (both expressed as mg/100 ml of serum) is greater than 70, then again calcium supplements should be omitted and in addition serum phosphorus levels should be carefully lowered by dietary restriction of protein phosphorus and by the use of oral aluminum gels.

In many patients with chronic renal failure, severe osteomalacia may develop because of the inability of the kidney to produce 1,25-dihydroxy-cholecalciferol (1,25-DHCC, the active form of vitamin D). Under these conditions, very large doses of vitamin D may have to be administered (about 50,000 to 100,000 IU/day). If this is done, serum calcium levels must be carefully monitored to prevent metastatic calcification. Recently, 1,25-DHCC has become available for experimental purposes and in microgram quantities appears able to slowly correct the low serum calcium levels and to reverse the osteomalacia, reduce the bone pain, and improve muscle power. The major advantage of the 1,25 compound is its short duration of action and hence its lack of storage in the body. If these good results continue, we can anticipate that 1,25-DHCC and its analog 1-α-hydroxycholecalciferol will soon be commercially available.

Recently, a modification of the diet outlined above has been under investigation. Instead of supplying the essential amino acids while restricting protein, this diet supplies the keto analogs of the essential amino acids while continuing to restrict protein. This diet is almost totally devoid of protein and relies on the body's ability to transaminate the keto acids into the essential amino acids. Hence, all of the nitrogen being utilized for protein turnover and for the synthesis of new protein comes from the body's elevated nonprotein nitrogen pool (mainly urea). Initial results with this approach have been very good. However, available evidence does not suggest any marked advantage in using this method over the method that supplies minimal amounts of essential amino acids. Since the latter is a less restrictive and a less expensive diet, it should continue to be used unless the use of keto analogs proves to give significantly better results.

Clearly the management of a patient with chronic renal failure requires a physician who can prescribe the exact type of diet required and a dietician with the skill and imagination to translate that diet into foods and meals that the patient will consume and can even enjoy. The Mayo Clinic has published exchange lists of foods for use by patients with chronic renal disease. They have also recently published a renal cookbook which is extremely useful to both dieticians and patients. In addition, most dieticians who work primarily with patients with renal disease have recipes of their own and exchange recipes with each other.

ACUTE RENAL FAILURE

In this symptom complex there is a sudden dramatic decrease in renal function and marked oliguria (less than 400 ml/day) which may persist for 2 weeks or longer. The disease most often occurs as a complication of surgery or trauma and can result in the patient's demise if it is not carefully managed. Initially, the patient is often unable to tolerate oral feedings. Because of fluid restriction (conditioned by the oliguria) the intake of calories and nutrients is almost always insufficient. During this period (usually 2 to 3 days) at least 100 g of glucose should be given as 500 ml of a 20% solution. If oral feedings cannot be begun after this period or if the BUN rises very rapidly, peritoneal dialysis or hemodialyis may have to be undertaken. As soon as oral feedings are feasible, the patient can be started on a diet similar to the kind recommended for chronic renal failure and uremia, 0.26 g of protein of high biologic value and 2000 to 3000 calories. In addition 20 meq of sodium, less than 45 meq of potassium, and no more than 750 to 1000 cc of fluid should be given. Hemodialysis should be used if the BUN continues to rise and to prevent hyperkalemia. A good rule to employ is to attempt to keep the BUN under 100 and to dialyze if it gets above that range. It should be pointed out that this type of diet, although mandatory and often life saving in a patient with acute renal failure, is often just the wrong type of diet for the patient's primary disease (trauma, surgery, burns, etc.), which often requires generous quantities of protein. Hence the diet should be instituted only if the patient demonstrates renal failure and should be continued only until renal function is recovered.

NEPHROTIC SYNDROME

This disease, both in adults and in children, is associated with massive proteinuria (more than 3.5 g/1.73 m^2/24 hr) and the presence of fat bodies in the urine. In addition, such patients often show hypoalbuminemia, hypercholesterolemia, hypertriglyceridemia, and edema which is often massive. The over-all dietary strategy depends on whether glomerular filtration rate (GFR), as measured by inulin or creatinine clearance, is significantly compromised. In cases where GFR is normal or nearly normal, the strategy is to replace the protein that is lost and to give some excess protein if possible. This is achieved in adults by prescribing high protein diets, 100 g/day or more, and adequate calories. Experience has shown that men may consume more than 120 g/day of protein for long periods. By contrast, women will rarely consume more than 100 g/day.

If the GFR is depressed, the regimen outlined in Table 1 should be undertaken. However, the daily protein intake should be increased by the amount lost in the urine and proteins of high biologic value should be used. At present, the significance of the high serum lipids in such patients with respect to atherosclerosis is unknown and hence clear recommendations about the intake of saturated fat and cholesterol cannot be made. From a practical standpoint, it is difficult to give a diet containing 100 g of protein, especially protein of high biologic value, while restricting saturated fat, and clearly the patient's present disease must take precedence over the theoretical possibility of preventing future disease. Again a skillful and imaginative dietician will play an essential role in translating 100 g of protein into enjoyable meals.

RENAL STONES

The management of the patient with renal stones often must employ modifications of diet, even though this condition is not strictly speaking due to renal disease. Central to all of the treatment, regardless of the nature of the stone or the metabolic abnormality that has led to stone formation, is the ingestion of large amounts of fluid. This is necessary because all of the types of stones result from an increased concentration of a particular substance in the urine. Simply diluting the urine, then, will reduce the concentration of the offending substance. Most individuals can be trained to drink 3 to 4 liters of fluid per day, which is the minimum these patients should consume. They should be instructed particularly to drink before going to bed at night and again when they get up to urinate. This is important because overnight urine tends normally to be concentrated. Patients who form stones should never be allowed to become dehydrated, and hence particular attention must be paid to hydration in hot climates or under conditions of strenuous exercise. On each visit to the physician, urine specific gravity should be checked. Some patients can be trained to do this at home. Since specific dietary and drug therapy will vary depending on the composition of the urinary stone, it is important that patients be instructed to collect any stones passed so that an accurate diagnosis can be made. Renal stones can be classified according to their chemical composition. The most common types are calcium stones, magnesium and ammonium phosphate stones, uric acid stones, and cystine stones.

Calcium Stones

Ninety percent of all renal stones in the United States are composed of calcium oxalate, calcium phosphate, or a mixture of both. Hyperparathyroidism is the most common disease that can result in formation of calcium stones. However, calcium stones may also appear as a complication of chronic small bowel disease, medullary sponge kidneys, renal tubular acidosis, sarcoidosis, hyperthyroidism, immobilization, calcium or vitamin D excess, urinary infection, Paget's disease, Cushing's syndrome, primary oxaluria, alkali abuse, and acetazolamide therapy. These conditions must therefore be ruled out when a calcium stone is passed. More common than all of these diseases combined is the patient who passes calcium stones for no apparent reason, or so-called idiopathic calcium stone disease. This syndrome accounts for about 70 to 80% of all cases of urolithiasis and probably represents several types of conditions that only recently are being defined. These include patients with idiopathic hypercalciuria, those with idiopathic hyperoxaluria, and others with no apparent abnormalities in either calcium or oxalate metabolism.

Normally, men excrete less than 300 to 400 mg/day of calcium in their urine and women excrete even less. In idiopathic hypercalciuria this level is exceeded and is accompanied by a normal serum calcium, a tendency toward reduced serum phosphate, and renal stone formation.

At the present time, the most effective therapy for patients with idiopathic hypercalciuria and renal calculi is restriction of calcium intake to 200 to 300 mg/day. (This can generally be accomplished by restricting milk and milk products and certain greens, such as collards and turnips.) In addition, medications containing calcium should not be taken and vitamin D itself or in fortified foods should be avoided. A high fluid intake, as was pointed out, is important and in addition hydrochlorothiazide, 50 mg twice daily, should be given. Some people also advocate reduced phosphate intake.

In patients with increased oxalate excretion in the urine either secondary to chronic small bowel disease in which oxalate absorption is increased, or due to yet undefined mechanisms, calcium oxalate stones may form. Certain vegetables (rhubarb, spinach, swiss chard, and beet roots), chocolate, and tea are rich in oxalate and should be restricted in any patient who has an elevated urinary oxalate excretion and has passed a calcium oxalate stone.

Magnesium Ammonium Phosphate Stones

These constitute about 10% of all stones and occur in patients with recurrent urinary infection involving urea splitting organisms. The ammonia thereby generated produces a highly alkaline urine in which magnesium ammonium phosphate precipitates in the form of crystals. The mainstay of therapy is permanent eradication of the infection. While this is being accomplished the urine can be acidified with 8 to 12 g/day of methionine or 500 mg of ascorbic acid several times per day. However, these agents should be used only for short periods of time and have only limited usefulness.

Uric Acid Stones

In patients with uric acid stones, the main aims are urinary dilution and alkalinization. Even if hyperuricemia is present, a low purine diet is generally not very effective in controlling stone formation. The mainstays of therapy are adequate fluid intake and the use of alkalinizing salt solutions to maintain urinary pH between 6 and 6.5. The most widely used solution is oral sodium citrate and citric acid in the form of Shohl's solution (1 ml forms 1 meq bicarbonate) given in a dosage of 10 to 30 ml or more after each meal, at bedtime, and in the middle of the night.

Cystine Stones

This rare type of renal stone occurs in patients with cystinuria who have a genetic defect in cystine, lysine, arginine, and ornithine transport in the GI tract and in the renal tubules. There is no effective dietary therapy. Fluid intake must be increased and urinary alkalinization is useful. In addition, if these measures are ineffective, a course of D-penicillamine can be instituted.

RECOMMENDED READING

Giovannetti, S., and Q. Maggiore, A Low-Nitrogen Diet with Proteins of High Biologic Value for Severe Chronic Uremia, *Lancet,* **1**, 1000 (1964).

Ing, T. S., and R. M. Kark, Renal Disease, in *Nutritional Support of Medical Practice,* H. A. Schneider, C. E. Anderson, and D. B. Coursin, Eds., Harper and Row, Hagerstown, Md., 1977, pp. 367–383.

Kopple, J. D. and J. W. Coburn, Metabolic Studies of Low Protein Diets in Uremia I. Nitrogen and Potassium, *Medicine,* **52**, 583 (1973), II Calcium, Phosphorus and Magnesium, *Medicine,* **52,** 597 (1973).

Kopple J. D., and M. E. Swendseid, Nitrogen Balance and Plasma Amino Acid Levels in Uremic Patients Fed an Essential Amino Acid Diet, *Am. J. Clin. Nutr.* **27**, 806 (1974).

Kopple, J. D., and M. E. Swendseid, Evidence that Histidine is an Essential Amino Acid in Normal and Chronically Uremic Man, *J. Clin. Invest.,* **55**, 881 (1975).

Thomas, W. C., Jr., Medical Aspects of Renal Calculous Disease, *Urol. Clinics North Amer.,* **1**, 261 (1974).

Varcoe, R., D. Halliday, E. R. Carson, P. Richards, and S. Tavill, Efficiency of Utilization of Urea Nitrogen for Albumin Synthesis by Chronically Uremic and Normal Men, *Clin. Sci. Molec. Med.,* **48**, 379 (1975).

Walser, M., A. W. Coulter, S. Dighe, and F. R. Cranty, The Effect of Keto-analogs of Essential Amino Acids in Severe Chronic Uremia, *J. Clin. Invest.,* **52**, 678 (1973).

21
DIABETES

Diabetes mellitus is the most common endocrine disease encountered in the United States and because of its morbidity and mortality it remains one of the most serious health problems in our society. Both from a physiologic and from a nutritional standpoint the disease may be viewed as two separate entities. In most cases, usually those beginning in middle age, although the absolute secretion of insulin is normal or even elevated, the end organ response to insulin is reduced, producing a *relative* insulin deficiency. In a smaller number of cases, usually beginning in childhood or adolescence, insulin secretion is low or absent and the patient suffers from an absolute deficiency of insulin.

From a therapeutic standpoint the aims in these two situations are considerably different. In the adult or maturity-onset diabetic the major aim of therapy is to restore conditions to a state in which the body becomes more responsive to insulin. If this can be accomplished the endogenous insulin, which is present in normal amounts, will be able to maintain carbohydrate homeostasis. Since the beta cells of the pancreas are able to respond to hyperglycemic stimuli and produce adequate amounts of insulin in maturity-onset diabetes, especially in the early stages, it is the response of the body to the released insulin that must be altered if the disease is to be reversed. By contrast, the juvenile diabetic must be treated with insulin, since the pancreas is unable to supply insulin in response to the usual stimulus. Hence the aim of therapy is to replace insulin in the most physiologic manner possible.

The nutrition of the patient is a crucial factor in both of these types of diabetes, but different types of dietary management must be employed in order to achieve the desired aim in each case.

MATURITY-ONSET DIABETES

Nutrition and Etiology

A great deal of evidence collected in the last 10 years strongly suggests that the risk of developing maturity-onset diabetes is influenced in a major way by nutritional factors. Changing dietary patterns in Japan, Israel, and Africa have been associated with a very great increase in the incidence of diabetes. Studies of aboriginal populations of the New World have demonstrated that the major changes that occurred in dietary habits and in exercise levels in these populations probably account for a tenfold increase in the incidence of diabetes. By contrast, studies in populations in which the prevalence of diabetes is usually high have demonstrated that during natural or imposed famine conditions both the appearance of new cases of diabetes and the severity of existing cases are reduced. For example, maturity-onset diabetes, a very common disease among Eastern European Jews, virtually disappeared during the imposed starvation in the Warsaw Ghetto during the early 1940s.

The nutritional factor that has shown the strongest and most consistent association with the prevalence of maturity-onset diabetes is the degree and duration of adiposity. There is little question that as a population gets fatter and as obesity persists within that population, more and more cases of diabetes appear. Clinical experience is certainly consistent with these observations. Maturity-onset diabetes, although not exclusively a disease of overweight people, is associated with increased adiposity in most cases. Since not all obese individuals get diabetes, the relationship between obesity and diabetes is a complicated one. There is no question that genetic factors strongly influence an individual's chances of becoming diabetic. Obesity seems to play its role by allowing the diabetic phenotype to express itself earlier and by increasing the severity of the disease. In addition, certain individuals who may be genetically at risk will develop the disease only if they are obese. People genetically not at risk presumably do not develop the disease even when they become obese.

It has been claimed that dietary sugar (monosaccharide and disaccharide) and fat are specifically diabetogenic. Several studies have shown that increased consumption of sugar, usually in the form of sucrose, has led to an increased incidence of diabetes. In these studies, however, almost invariably the intake of total calories has increased. Within a given population there does not seem to be an association between incidence of diabetes and previous sugar consumption. Moreover, diabetics were not found to have previously consumed more sugar than nondiabetics. By contrast, within these same populations, obesity was always much more common among diabetics.

The consumption of large amounts of fat or large amounts of refined sugar by a population almost invariably means that that population is consuming too many calories. This is certainly true in most westernized countries today. Sugar is a pleasant, low bulk way of insidiously ingesting calories. Fat is the nutrient highest in calories. Most evidence would implicate calories, not their source, as the major dietary factor contributing to the high rates of diabetes in our society.

The mechanisms by which obesity leads to increased rates of diabetes are not clearly understood. Animal experiments have shown that obesity is associated with resistance to endogenous insulin. Moreover, since insulin is very important in regulating turnover rates of lipid derived from the adipose depot, the larger the adipose depot the greater the demand on the pancreas. If an individual is genetically prone to develop diabetes, it seems reasonable to assume that the prolonged strain on the beta cells imposed by chronic obesity may lead to the expression of the disease. In this regard, the effect of repeated weight loss and weight gain over a prolonged period is not known. It is conceivable that such a chain of events might even place a greater strain on the pancreas than obesity itself.

The lack of clear association between sugar and fat intake and the incidence of diabetes should not confuse the need to reduce the intake of these components in the management of diabetes. As we shall see, control of certain diabetics is much more easily attained when the intake of refined sugars is curtailed, and complications of diabetes may be averted if the intake of fat, particularly animal fat, is lowered.

Complications

Before discussing the nutritional management of the individual with maturity-onset diabetes, it is important to review the complications of diabetes and the relation of these complications to diet. It is the complications and not the disease itself which for the vast majority of diabetics are most life threatening. Among different populations of diabetics major differences in the frequency of certain complications have been noted. In Japan, for example, the incidence of coronary artery disease and peripheral vascular disease among diabetics is much lower than it is in the United States. The best explanation for the relatively low rates of atherosclerosis and its complications seen in diabetics in many Asian, African, and South American countries is the lower consumption in these countries of cholesterol and saturated fat (both before and after the discovery of diabetes). In addition, caloric intake in relation to energy expenditure is usually lower in these populations. This is not to say that diabetics in these countries are not more prone to atherosclerosis and its complications than the general population; they are. However since diabetes is only one of several risk factors for developing atherosclerosis, and since these risk factors are additive, the appearance of atherosclerosis is much more likely to occur in diabetics who are more at risk from other factors. In this respect, serum lipid levels in the general population seem to be the most important factor and these levels are related to dietary intake of saturated fat and cholesterol. However, the lower incidence of hypertension and cigarette smoking in some of these populations may also contribute to the lower incidence of atherosclerosis among diabetics.

In general, geographic and ethnic differences are much less common in respect to the second major group of long-term diabetic complications, small-vessel disease or microvascular disease (glomerulosclerosis and retinopathy). Even here, however, there are a few societies, such as the Navajo Indian and the Nigerian, in which the incidence of these complications is considerably reduced. Whether nutritional factors are involved is at present unknown and should be investigated. Another complication, acidosis and ketosis, also seems to vary among different populations of diabetics. Again it is unclear what relation, if any, nutritional factors may play in this variation.

Diet Therapy

It should be clear from the above discussion that the major aim of dietary therapy in the patient with maturity-onset diabetes is the reduction of adiposity. Weight reduction by restricting calories or by increasing exercise or both will reduce hyperglycemia. More important these measures, when successful, will reduce the insulin resistance which accompanies obesity. This will reduce the stress on the pancreas and will usually result in a significant improvement in beta cell function. Thus diet, specifically a reducing diet, in this group will not only help to control the disease but also reduces its severity. The return of blood glucose levels to normal and complete reversal of the glucose tolerance test to a normal pattern as a result of a reducing regimen alone is uncommon, largely because achieving and maintaining optimal body weight are rare. Nevertheless even partial reduction of adiposity is helpful. The type of reducing diet employed is particularly important when dealing with the overweight diabetic. Most of the crash diets, which tend to be nutritionally inbalanced, are contraindicated in the treatment of diabetics. For example, the Atkins diet leads to ketosis and hyperlipidemia, two complications particularly dangerous in diabetes. The high protein diets all impose an added burden on the kidney, which again may be dangerous in a patient with diabetes. Diets that concentrate on fruits may be particularly high in simple sugars and hence impose an added strain on the beta cells. Thus a balanced reduction in caloric intake is by far the best approach to weight reduction in the individual with diabetes. Crash programs of any type should not be used. The use of exchange foods as outlined in Chapter 12 for weight reduction is a particularly practical approach in managing the diabetic patient because, as we shall see, the dietary management of most diabetics also involves a qualitative change in the components of the diet. At any given level of calories this can be done by using the same exchange lists. In fact, the exchange list recommended in Chapter 12 for obesity is the same list employed by the American Diabetes Association for managing patients with diabetes. Hence, by employing this approach, a simple and practical diabetic dietary regimen can be constructed at any caloric intake.

Just as weight reduction is the main nutritional consideration in the control of diabetes, reduction of saturated fat and cholesterol, especially in the western societies, is the main nutritional consideration in prevention of the atherosclerotic complications of the disease. Thus, in my judgment, all patients who have diabetes should be placed on a prudent diet, limiting cholesterol intake to 300 mg/day and reducing saturated fat while increasing polyunsaturated fat intake. Again, the exchange tables recommended in Chapter 12 are useful, and the same advice given to any patient with hyperlipidemia can be given to the diabetic patient.

If weight reduction can be accomplished to the extent of complete reversal of diabetic symptoms and a return of the glucose tolerance test to normal, no further dietary manipulation is necessary other than maintaining the patient at this optimal weight. Since this kind of complete reversal is not usually achieved, many experts recommend a diet which is not only restricted in calories but which is also aimed at placing a minimum strain on the already overtaxed islets. To this end they suggest restriction or complete avoidance of refined sugars, and of certain naturally occurring monosaccharides and disaccharides. Although I am not convinced that there is much benefit to be derived from this approach in diabetic patients who do not require insulin, it is a relatively simple matter, using the exchange tables, to avoid certain foods that are high in refined sugar. Another type of control that is often imposed is an attempt to establish new eating patterns in the patient with diabetes. A certain consistency in the quantity, quality, and timing of the meals in obese diabetics is often advised. This, of course, may be desirable to some extent in any obese patient, but it is not a major concern in the obese diabetic. In fact, studies suggest that a high degree of consistency is not necessary on a daily basis in the amount of calories, starch, or other nutrients consumed, or in the timing of feedings as long as the long-term ingestion of calories is low enough to control adiposity. Between meal and bedtime snacks are not necessary and are often counterproductive in the obese diabetic.

Some patients will not be brought under acceptable control by using dietary management alone and will require insulin as well. In such patients, the use of between meal and prebedtime snacks may be of some value in avoiding rapid changes in blood sugar levels. However, the calories in these snacks must be calculated into the total daily caloric allotment for the particular patient. In such a patient, simple sugars, especially taken alone, are to be avoided since they are rapidly absorbed and will induce rapid changes in blood sugar. This, in turn, places an added burden on the pancreatic beta cells, which presumably are already working at maximum output. As a result, hyperglycemia may be prolonged and postprandial drops in blood sugar may be deeper than normal.

JUVENILE-ONSET DIABETES

In contrast to maturity-onset diabetes, the juvenile variety is characterized by an absolute insulin deficiency. The most current information suggests that the disease is the result of a viral infection, which in certain individuals of a particular isoantigenic makeup produces specific destruction of the pancreatic beta cells. The disease is not usually associated with obesity and because of the weight loss that often accompanies the disease before it is discovered these patients are often underweight. The course of the disease during its early stages is often quite rapid, the patient progressing from polyurea, polydipsia, and weight loss in spite of an increased appetite to a state of ketoacidosis and eventual diabetic coma. The treatment always involves the use of insulin, which must be sustained throughout the patient's life. The use of diet in this disease is as an adjunct to insulin therapy but is very important in maintaining proper control. In these patients calories should not be restricted below normal levels. Meals should be smaller and one to three between meal snacks should be taken to roughly match the time-action pattern of administered insulin. This type of feeding pattern will blunt postprandial rises in blood sugar and protect against hypoglycemia, since no endogenous insulin is available in response to meals. These patients require much more constancy of meal patterns, distribution, and actual dietary makeup than obese maturity-onset diabetics. In addition, they need to be advised how best to deal with situations that invariably will occur, such as delay in a meal, unusual exercise, or complicating illness.

In both types of diabetes restricting carbohydrates is no longer emphasized because insulin requirement has been shown to be more related to the total fuel supply than to the fuel source. The liver is quite capable of converting both complex carbohydrates and amino acids into glucose. A number of clinical studies have demonstrated that diets which contain generous amounts of starch are well tolerated by both insulin-dependent and insulin-independent diabetics. Simple sugars should be curtailed in the insulin-dependent individual to prevent marked swings in blood sugar postprandially. It is worth noting that recent evidence suggests that the ingestion of high amounts of fiber may slow down monosaccharide absorption from the gut and thereby blunt the expected sharp rise in blood sugar. Even patients with type IV lipoproteinemia will tolerate starch well as long as levels of dietary sugar and total calories are appropriately controlled.

A second reason for not restricting carbohydrate intake is that to impose such a restriction and still keep total calories adequate the diet must be relatively high in fat and cholesterol. Because the major complication in both types of diabetics is atherosclerosis, such a diet is not desirable. In the past when carbohydrate was restricted the typical diet for diabetics in America consisted of about 42% of calories from fat and was very high in cholesterol. In North American diabetics controlled on this type of diet, coronary artery disease was very common and indeed was the major cause of death. By contrast, diabetics maintained on high carbohydrate, low fat, low cholesterol diets had a much lower incidence of coronary artery disease. These considerations have led most physicians who treat large numbers of people with diabetes to prescribe diets that contain more starch and less saturated fat and cholesterol than previously. In addition to the added starch, the calories that must be replaced from the lowering in animal fat can come from two other sources, vegetable fat and protein. Thus a typeical modern diabetic diet will have the following characteristics:

1. Calories should be adequate to reach or maintain optimum weight.
2. Refined sugars should be absent or sharply limited. Ten to 15% of calories should be from natural sugars (fruit, vegetables, milk).
3. Fat should be limited to 25 to 35% of calories.
4. Saturated fat supplies 10 to 15% of calories ($\frac{1}{2}$ typical American diet); vegetable fat (monounsaturated and polyunsaturated) supplies about 15 to 20% of calories.
5. Protein can range from 12 to 24% of calories (not critical). Children and pregnant or lactating women require at least 1.5 g/kg.
6. The remainder of calories (30 to 40%) should come from complex carbohydrates (usually starch).

Diabetes

Although there are a number of ways to formulate such a diet, the use of exchange tables is simple and effective and has the advantage of allowing the patient maximum flexibility. Table 1 is an abbreviated form of the exchange lists employed by the American Diabetic Association. Within each category, one food can be exchanged for another and in certain situations food can be exchanged between categories. (However, this is more difficult, because these foods usually differ qualitatively in their nutrient content).

The first consideration in planning the diet is to determine the patient's eating habits and food preferences. Almost all diabetic diets can be tailored

Table 1.   Food exchange lists

List 1. Free Foods

Boullion	Gelatin,	Mustard	Chicory	Lettuce
Clear broth	unsweetened	Pickle, sour	Chinese cabbage	(all kinds)
Coffee	Lemon, lime	Pickle, dill—un-	Endive	Parsley
Tea		sweetened	Escarole	Radishes
		Vinegar		Watercress

List 2. Vegetable Exchanges = $^1/_2$ Cup Cooked or 1 Cup Raw

Asparagus	Carrots	Mushrooms	Tomatoes
Bean sprouts	Catsup (2 tbsp.)	Okra	1 cup raw;
Beans (green or	Cauliflower	Onions	$^1/_2$ cup cooked
wax)	Celery	Peppers (red or	Tomato or vege-
Broccoli	Cucumbers	green)	table juice—6 oz.
Beets	Eggplant	Rutabaga	All leafy greens
Brussels sprouts		Sauerkraut	
Cabbage		Summer squash	
(all kinds)			

List 3. Fruit Exchanges

FRUITS   JUICES

Apple—$^1/_2$ med.	Cantaloupe—$^1/_4$	Mango—	Peach—1 med.	Apple, Pine-
Applesauce—	med. (6″ dia.)	$^1/_2$ small	Pear—1 small	apple—$^1/_3$ cup
$^1/_2$ cup	Cherries—10	Nectarine—	Pineapple—	Grapefruit,
Apricots, fresh—	large	1 small	$^1/_2$ cup	orange—$^1/_2$
2 med.	Dates—2	Orange—	Prunes, dried—2	cup
Apricots, dried—	Figs, dried—1	1 small	Raisins—2 tbsp.	Grape, prune—
4 halves	small	Papaya—	Strawberries—	$^1/_4$ cup
Bananas—$^1/_2$	Fruit cocktail,	$^1/_3$ med.	$^3/_4$ cup	
small	canned—$^1/_2$ cup		Tangerine—1	
Blueberries—$^1/_2$	Grapefruit—$^1/_2$		large	
cup	small		Watermelon—1	
	Grapes—12		cup cubed	
	Honeydew			
	melon—$^1/_3$ (7″			
	dia.)			

Table 1. (*Continued*)

List 4. Starch Exchanges (Cooked Servings)

BREADS	CRACKERS	CEREALS	VEGETABLES	ALCOHOL
Any loaf—1 slice	Graham ($2^{1}/_2''$ sq.)—2	Hot cereal—$^{1}/_2$ cup	Beans or peas (plain) cooked— $^{1}/_2$ cup	Beer—5 oz.
Bagel—$^{1}/_2$	Matzoh ($4'' \times 6''$)—$^{1}/_2$	Dry flakes—$^{2}/_3$ cup	Corn—$^{1}/_3$ cup or $^{1}/_2$ med. ear.	Whiskey—1 oz.
Dinner roll—1 ($2''$ dia.)	Melba toast—4	Dry puffed—$1^{1}/_2$ cups	Parsnips— $^{2}/_3$ cup	Wine, dry— $2^{1}/_2$ oz.
English muffin—$^{1}/_2$	Oysters ($^{1}/_2$ cup)—20	Bran—5 tbsp.	Potatoes, white— 1 small or $^{1}/_2$ cup	Wine, sweet— $1^{1}/_2$ oz.
Bun, hamburger or hotdog—$^{1}/_2$	Pretzels—8 rings	Wheatgerm— 2 tbsp.	Potatoes, sweet or yams—$^{1}/_4$ cup	
Cornbread ($1^{1}/_2''$)—1 cube	Rye krisps—3	Pastas—$^{1}/_2$ cup	Pumpkin—$^{3}/_4$ cup	
Tortilla ($6''$ dia.)—1	Saltines—5	Rice—$^{1}/_2$ cup	Winter squash— $^{1}/_2$ cup	

DESSERTS

Fat-free sherbet—
4 oz.
Angel cake—
$1^{1}/_2''$ square

List 5. Meat Exchanges (Cooked weight)

Beef, dried, chipped— 1 oz.	Poultry without skin—1 oz.	Lobster—1 small tail	Egg—1 med.
Beef, lamb, pork, veal lean only— 1 oz.	Fish—1 oz.	Oysters, clams, shrimp— 5 med.	Hard cheese—$^{1}/_2$ oz.
Cottage cheese, uncreamed— $^{1}/_4$ cup		Tuna, packed in water—$^{1}/_4$ cup	Peanut butter— 2 tsp.
		Salmon, pink, canned—$^{1}/_4$ cup	

List 6. Milk Exchanges

Buttermilk, fat free—1 cup	Skim milk—1 cup
Yogurt, plain, made with nonfat milk— $^{3}/_4$ cup	1% fat milk—7 oz.

List 7. Fat Exchanges

Avocado ($4''$ dia.)—$^{1}/_8$	French dressing—1 tbsp.	Roquefort dressing— 2 tsp.	Peanuts—10
Bacon, crisp—1 slice	Mayonnaise— 1 tsp.	Thousand Island dressing— 2 tsp.	Walnuts—6 small
Butter, margarine—1 tsp.		Oil—1 tsp.	
		Olives—5 small	

to respect these preferences. Second, the total number of calories to be consumed should be set. This will depend on the patient's degree of adiposity, the age, height, and weight of the patient, and his activity. Third, the number of feedings to be used should be decided on. This will vary with the type of diabetic patient. In general, maturity-onset diabetics not requiring insulin can do well on three meals. In the mild insulin-stable diabetic who is receiving insulin a small midmorning snack may be employed, especially for a patient who consumes a very small breakfast. Similarly, a late evening snack may be desirable if the patient had a light or early dinner. In the severe insulin-dependent diabetic, calorie intake should be distributed throughout the day, usually among three meals and two to three snacks, depending on when and in what form the insulin is given. Since most of these patients are lean and are not being restricted in calories, this type of spacing offers no special problems. Fourth, the percentage of each of the major nutrients is set forth. Most diets should follow the guidelines above. However, with those guidelines there is still room for a wide variety of menu plans. At this point, the dietician, who has been working with the physician from the onset, can translate the diet prescription into a variety of menu plans. If these principles are employed successfully, the patient should be on a diet that is appropriate in calories for the desired objective, low in animal fat and cholesterol, relatively high in polyunsaturated fat, high in carbohydrate but low in simple sugars, and if insulin is being used, properly spaced throughout the day to minimize wide spreads in blood sugar levels. Table 2 compares the typical American diet with the diabetic diets recommended here.

Certain special dietary concerns should be anticipated and discussed with the patient. For example, if a meal must be delayed in an insulin-

Table 2. Distribution of major nutrients (% calories)

	Starch and Other Polysaccharides	Sugars	Fat	Protein	Alcohol
Typical American diet	25–35	30	35–45 ($^2/_3$ sat.)	12–19	0–10
Diabetic diet	35–45	5–15[a]	25–35 (less than $^1/_2$ sat.)	12–24	0–6

[a] Almost exclusively natural sugars mainly in fruit and milk.

dependent diabetic, a carbohydrate snack from those which are permissible should be eaten. The same is true if the patient is to be engaged in exercise that is much greater than usual. The question of artificial sweeteners and dietetic foods will almost always come up. They are certainly not necessary in the adequate feeding of a patient with diabetes. However, they can be used as long as their actual nutrient content is calculated into the daily diet. For the obese diabetic with a sweet tooth, they may be useful. In general, however, it is unwise for the patient to become dependent on the use of these sweeteners.

It is unfortunate that successful dietary management in patients with diabetes is not as common as it should be. The reasons for this sad state of affairs are that patients often do not understand the dietary advice, physicians are unable to give proper dietary advice, physicians and dieticians still cling to limiting carbohydrate and hence give diets high in fat, diets are prescribed which are difficult for the patient to follow, and a host of others. Whatever the reasons, we can do better. To this end we must educate ourselves, communicate with our patients, and work closely with other professionals who can help us translate our nutritional goals into wholesome and exciting meal plans.

RECOMMENDED READING

Anderson, J. W., and R. H. Herman, Effects of Carbohydrate Restriction on Glucose Tolerance of Normal Men and Reactive Hypoglycemic Patients, *Am. J. Clin. Nutr.*, **28**, 748 (1975).

Bierman, E. L., M. J. Albrink, R. A. Arky, W. E. Connor, S. Dayton, N. Spritz, and D. Steinberg, Special Report: Principles of Nutrition and Dietary Recommendations for Patients with Diabetes Mellitus, *Diabetes*, **20**, 633–634 (1971).

Brunzell, J. D., R. L. Lerner, W. R. Hazzard, D. Porte, Jr., and E. L. Bierman, Improved Glucose Tolerance with High Carbohydrate Feeding in Mild Diabetes, *N. Engl. J. Med.*, **284**, 521 (1971).

Brunzell, J. D., R. L. Lerner, D. Porte, Jr., and E. L. Bierman, Effect of a Fat Free High Carbohydrate Diet on Diabetic Subjects with Fasting Hyperglycemia, *Diabetes*, **23**, 138 (1974).

Christakis, G., and A. Miridjanian, The Nutritional Aspects of Diabetes, in M. Ellenberg and M. Rifkin, Eds., *Diabetes Mellitus: Theory and Practice*, McGraw-Hill, New York, 1970, p. 594.

Krall, L. P. and A. P. Joslin, General Plan of Treatment and Diet Regulation, in A. Marble, Ed., *Joslin's Diabetes Mellitus*, 11th ed., Lea and Febiger, Philadelphia, 1971, pp. 832–857.

Schmitt, D. B., An Argument for the Unmeasured Diet in Juvenile Diabetes, *Clin. Pediat.*, **14**, 68 (1975).

West, K. M., Diabetes Mellitus, in H. A. Schneider, C. E. Anderson, and D. B. Coursin, Eds., *Nutritional Support of Medical Practice*, Harper and Row, Hagerstown, Md., 1977.

Wood, F. C., Jr., and E. L. Bierman, New Concepts in Diabetic Dietetics, *Nutr. Today*, **7**, 4 (1972).

22

ENTERAL AND PARENTERAL NUTRITION

ENTERAL NUTRITION AND DEFINED FORMULA DIETS

Under certain conditions patients cannot consume amounts of normal foods adequate to meet their requirements. Such patients must be supplemented with artificially prepared mixtures either by mouth, if this route is feasible, or by nasogastric, gastrostomy, or jejunostomy tube if these are indicated. Among the most important indications for this type of management are:

1. Any severe illness that increases nutrient requirements (fever, sepsis, cancer, trauma, burns, surgery, etc.) and at the same time reduces appetite and renders the patient too weak to ingest sufficient food.
2. Unconscious or delirious patients unable to feed themselves or swallow properly.
3. Cancer or any other disease that obstructs the upper alimentary tract.

Oral Supplements

Oral supplements should be used in patients who can consume foods by mouth but require such foods in a particular consistency or who require supplementation because they are unable to consume adequate calories and protein from a regular diet. The basic principle is to supply a concentrated source of calories and protein in an easily ingested, palatable form. Proprietary preparations, usually prepared from casein and fat, are

236

on the market and can be mixed readily with other foods, increasing the over-all caloric and protein content of the diet. These preparations can be mixed with vegetable oil and sugar or dextrose in any proportion and various flavoring agents can be added. Varying amounts of water can be added and different consistencies can thus be obtained. Such mixtures can be served as hot or cold drinks, as ice-cream, as puddings, and, if a little gelatin is added, as a jelly. With an imaginative dietary staff able to prepare novel preparations and to encourage patient cooperation, adequate quantities of such concentrated foods can often be consumed by patients convalescing from severe illnesses or surgical procedures.

Nasogastric Feeding

Complete nutrition can be supplied through a nasogastric tube. Such feedings can be supplied in the form of natural foodstuffs blended to liquid consistency or as prepared mixtures of nutrients. Large amounts of fluids may be administered by this route, which may be particularly important in the dehydrated patient. In addition, food supplements and medications, which may be distasteful to the patient, can be given directly through the tube. Once it is in position, there is little discomfort and the patient is able to sleep comfortably with the tube in place, to cough and discharge oral secretions, and to ingest food orally if this is desired. The tube should be removed every 48 hours and a new tube passed through the opposite nostril. There are certain situations which preclude the use of nasogastric feedings. These include:

1. Lesions of the mouth, pharynx, or esophagus.
2. Patients with cuffed endotracheal tubes or tracheostomies.
3. Vomiting.
4. Inability of the lower GI tract to tolerate any feedings.

Initially 50 cc of water should be administered through the tube. After 1 hour the stomach is aspirated to make sure the water is no longer present. Subsequently the actual feedings are begun in small volume and strength. These are gradually increased to the desired amount and nutrient content over a 24 to 48 hour period. It is essential to aspirate the tube before each feeding to be sure it is still in the stomach. The total amount of fluid in an adult should be around 2 liters in a 24 hour period. This amount may be increased if the patient is dehydrated or has excessive fluid loss that must be replaced. A number of preparations can be made up using milk, eggs, vegetable oil, sucrose, or dextrose, or employing diluted blended mixtures of other foods. Caloric requirements and requirements for protein and other nutrients will depend on the patient's age, sex, size, and medical condition. There are several proprietary mixtures available which can be used for nasogastric feeding. If these are used, the physician must be sure that the formula chosen meets the requirements of the patient. This must be ascertained not only for calories, protein, and fat, but for vitamins and minerals as well. If necessary any of the commercially available enteral feedings can be supplemented with other nutrients. Almost any type of diet, low salt, low fat, high carbohydrate–low protein, can be given through a nasogastric tube by blending the desired ingredients to the proper consistency and suitably diluting them with water. In certain situations, mainly those involving disease processes within the gastrointestinal tract, dilute solutions may be necessary. This is particularly true if diarrhea is present. Sometimes feeding by slow drip over a prolonged period will allow such patients to tolerate enteral feeding better than giving the daily requirement in three to four separate "meals." In patients with steatorrhea medium-chain triglycerides may be substituted for the usual vegetable oil emulsions.

Gastrostomy and Jejunostomy Feeding

The principles are the same as with nasogastric feedings and the general indications are the same. If nasogastric intubation is possible it is the route of choice. However, when this route cannot be used, for example, because of disease in the esophagus, a tube can be surgically placed in the stomach. Under certain situations, especially when the stomach is diseased, a tube may be inserted surgically into the duodenum for feeding purposes. The actual feedings used are similar to those employed in nasogastric feedings and must be modified according to the patient's primary disease.

PARENTERAL NUTRITION

Situations may occur in clinical practice in which, for a variety of reasons, the patient cannot be fed through the gastrointestinal tract. In the past such patients could be maintained for only relatively short periods by supplying intravenous calories and minimal amounts of nitrogen, usually in the form of glucose and protein hydrolysates. The actual nutritional requirements of the patient could not be met using this approach, and if oral or tube feedings could not be started relatively soon, deterioration, progressive emaciation, and death ensued. In the 1950s attempts were made to introduce the use of intravenous fat emulsions to increase the number of calories that could be administered. Unfortunately the experience with the preparations available at that time was very poor and so many severe toxic reactions were reported that the intravenous use of lipids was abandoned. In the late 1960s the concept of using hypertonic solutions of glucose together with protein hydrolysates or crystalline amino acids was introduced by Dudrick at the University of Pennsylvania. To accomplish this, however, a safe method for inserting a catheter into a central vein (usually the superior or inferior vena cava) had to be devised because these hypertonic solutions rapidly sclerosed peripheral veins. This method made it possible for the first time to maintain patients for long periods on total parenteral feedings. Shortly after this method began to be employed clinically, Wretlind reintroduced the use of intravenous lipid emulsions in Europe. Using a soy bean oil and egg yolk phospholipid preparation (Intralipid), he was able to feed patients by the intravenous route without the toxic reactions of the previously used fat preparations. The use of intravenous fat made more complete nutrition available to the patient and also made possible the use of either peripheral or central veins (since less hypertonic solutions could be employed). Thus at present it is possible to maintain patients for long periods of time without any food passing through the GI tract. In fact, with the use of these techniques, patients are being maintained at home for long periods (some for several years). They have been taught to mix and administer their own solutions, usually through a catheter which has been inserted into the superior vena cava and tunneled through the skin to an accessible site. Although these developments have opened a new and exciting era in the treatment of a variety of diseases, they have also highlighted perhaps more than any other clinical situation the necessity for understanding the basic principles of nutrition. For now, for the first time, precise nutrients were being used and diets were being formulated by mixing solutions that had to contain the proper number of nutrients in the proper proportions. For total parenteral nutrition to be successfully used, the solutions must contain proper amounts of water, electrolytes, and other minerals, water-soluble and fat-soluble vitamins, as well as calories derived from carbohydrate and fat and nitrogen from protein.

Amino Acids

Table 1 lists the amino acids that should be available in any solution to be used for total parenteral nutrition and the reasons for their use.

The eight essential amino acids cannot be synthesized by adult man and hence must be supplied. In addition, cysteine-cystine cannot be synthesized in sufficient quantity from methionine in the fetus and premature infant, and in the adult, although deficiency symptoms do not develop

Table 1.   Amino acid constituents of parenteral solutions.

Amino Acid	Reason for Use
Isoleucine, leucine, lysine, methionine, phenylalanine, threonine, tryptophan, valine	Essential under all circumstances
Arginine	Essential for optimal utilization of amino acid mixtures and for detoxification
Cysteine-cystine	Essential for the fetus. Necessary to maintain normal cystine blood levels in the adult
Histidine	Essential for infants and in uremia
Tyrosine	Essential for premature infants
Alanine, glutamic acid, proline	Necessary for optimal utilization of amino acid mixtures
Aspartic acid, glycine serine	Sources of nonspecific nitrogen

in their absence, their concentration in blood drops when they are not supplied. Since phenylalanine cannot be adequately converted to tyrosine in prematures, solutions without tyrosine, when used in premature infants, result in a drop in the tyrosine level in the blood. Histidine is also essential for infants and in addition may be necessary for optimal utilization of the amino acid mixture in patients with uremia.

Arginine, although not an essential amino acid, can be synthesized in only limited quantities by the body. Therefore, it must be supplied if optimum utilization of the amino acid mixture is to be obtained. Moreover, arginine counteracts certain toxic effects that are produced when glycine is used in larger amounts. Clinical data suggest also that alanine, glutamic acid, and proline are necessary for optimal utilization. The aspartic acid, glycine, and serine are used as nonspecific nitrogen sources.

The minimum daily requirements of the eight essential amino acids for an adult are shown in Table 2.

Thus any solution designed to provide total nutrition must contain at least these amounts of essential amino acids. In practice, considerably more is usually given.

Not only are the absolute amounts of essential amino acids crucial but the proportion of essential amino acids (E) to total nitrogen (T) is also important. The E:T ratio (grams of essential amino acids per gram of total nitrogen) is usually about 3 in proteins of high biologic value (egg 3.2), and 2 or below in proteins of low biologic value. Thus a well-designed

Table 2.   Adult minimum daily requirements

Amino Acid	Requirement (g/day)
Isoleucine	0.7
Leucine	1.1
Lysine	0.8
Methionine	1.1 (up to 30% can be replaced by cystine-cysteine)
Phenylalanine	1.1 (up to 50% can be replaced by tyrosine)
Threonine	0.5
Tryptophan	0.25
Valine	0.8

intravenous solution should contain both essential and nonessential amino acids in such quantities as to achieve an E:T ratio of about 3. In addition, proteins of high biologic value usually contain close to 50% of their amino acid composition as essential amino acids (egg 46%). Approximating this proportion is desirable in the solutions to be employed. The most widely used protein hydrolysate, Aminosol, and the two most widely used mixtures of crystalline amino acids, FreAmine II (United States) and Vamin (Sweden), are all very close to the desired proportions. However, in some countries products that are not mixed in these desirable proportions are used.

Administered amino acids are optimally utilized only when the solution contains adequate calories in the proper form and when adequate amounts of other nutrients are given. Table 3 lists the most favorable conditions for amino acid utilization.

Table 3.   Fundamentals of parenteral solutions

1. Adequate amounts of amino acids
   Adults—above 0.7 g/kg/day
   Infants—above 2.5 g/kg/day
2. E:T about 3
3. 45 to 50% of total nitrogen in the form of essential amino acids
4. Adequate energy supply (150 to 200 kcal/g nitrogen)
5. At least 20% of calories from carbohydrate
6. Simultaneous supply of amino acids and energy
7. Adequate supply of other nutrients

Carbohydrates

Carbohydrate is given mainly in the form of glucose, with smaller amounts of fructose used in certain centers. Until 1975 in the United States, intravenous fat emulsions were not commercially available and highly concentrated glucose solutions, 20 to 40%, had to be used to supply calories in the range of 2000 to 3000 per day. There are some studies which suggest that the use of invert sugar in solutions cantaining 10% glucose and 10% fructose might have some advantages over 20% glucose solutions.

With the introduction of intravenous lipid, it is no longer necessary to give sugar solutions of such high concentrations. About 200 to 250 g/day of glucose can be supplied easily by using a 10% solution. This, when given together with the amino acids, will supply 800 to 1000 calories and will promote optimal utilization. In addition, such solutions may be administered either through a peripheral or a central catheter. The remaining calories can be given as a fat emulsion (20%), 500 cc of which will supply about 900 calories. Thus, a total of about 2000 to 2500 calories can be given in 2500 cc of fluid in this manner. Such a solution gives about 10 to 13% of the energy from protein (amino acids), 50% from carbohydrate, and 40% from fat, not unlike many natural diets.

Fat Emulsions

Intravenous fat is used primarily for two purposes: to make calories available in a concentrated form and to supply essential fatty acids. There are several studies demonstrating that administration of the soybean oil, egg yolk phospholipid emulsion Intralipid, in quantities making up about 40% of calories, is safe and produces no major side effects, and that the fat is well utilized. Even as much as 200 g of fat (3 g/kg), or 60 to 80% of calories, has been given safely. At present, about 2 g/kg, or about 40% of the total daily caloric intake, is recommended. In infants the recommendation would be about 2.5 to 3g/kg/day, or even slightly more.

One of the complications of total parenteral nutrition prior to the use of intravenous fat was essential fatty acid deficiency (see Chapter 7). In adults, a characteristic dermatitis has been found which disappears when intravenous lipid is administered. The requirement for essential fatty acid has not been definitely determined, and estimates of adult requirements range from 7.5 to 25 g/day. Hence only 0.1 to 0.3 g/kg/day of linoleic acid is required, and this amount is present in 15 g of soybean oil, which is the main constituent of Intralipid. Essential fatty acid deficiency is more common in infants maintained on intravenous feedings without fat. In infants 3 to 4% of energy intake should be supplied as linoleic acid. This amounts to around 0.4 g/kg/day of linoleic acid.

Vitamins and Minerals

The requirements for all vitamins and minerals must be met in patients receiving intravenous nutrition. Table 4 sets forth the daily recommended allowances for vitamins in adults and infants. These quantities must be considered tentative since careful studies to determine intravenous vitamin requirements are still in progress.

The water-soluble vitamins are added to the solutions containing glucose and amino acids and the fat-soluble vitamins to the intravenous lipid solution. Particular attention must be paid to vitamin K. As pointed out in Chapter 8 vitamin K is formed by intestinal bacteria in most healthy adults and hence is not required to be supplied in the diet. However, patients on antibiotics who were receiving intravenous nutrition without vitamin K have developed deficiency symptoms with severe and even fatal bleeding within 9 days. Presumably this situation is due to a change in the intestinal flora and decreased vitamin K production. Thus, vitamin K, as well as other vitamins, should always be given daily to every patient on intravenous alimentation. Recently, it has been noted that some patients on home parenteral nutrition for long periods of time have developed

Table 4. Tentative recommended daily allowances

	Adult (amt/kg/day)	Neonate and Infant (amt/kg/day)
Water-soluble vitamins		
Thiamin	0.02 mg	0.05 mg
Riboflavin	0.03 mg	0.1 mg
Nicotinamide	0.2 mg	1 mg
Pyridoxine	0.03 mg	0.1 mg
Folic acid	3.0 μg	20.0 μg
B_{12}	0.03 μg	0.2 μg
Pantothenic acid	0.2 mg	1.0 mg
Biotin	5.0 μg	30.0 μg
Ascorbic acid	0.5 mg	3.0 mg
Fat-soluble vitamins		
Retinol (A)	10 μg	0.1 mg
Vitamin D	0.04 μg	2.5 μg
Vitamin K	2 μg	50 μg
Vitamin E	1.5 mg	3 mg

signs of vitamin A deficiency. This has been traced to the fact that vitamin A may cling to the bag that is used for administering the intravenous solutions. Studies are under way to find a way to correct this problem.

Intravenous solutions containing sodium, potassium, magnesium, calcium, and chloride have been in use for a long time. However, other essential minerals must be supplied if total intravenous nutrition is being employed. The exact requirements for the various trace minerals are still being determined. Phosphorus and zinc seem to be of special importance. Adult patients being maintained on total intravenous nutrition with solutions lacking phosphate were shown to be significantly hypophosphatemic within 7 to 10 day. The reduced amount of 2,3-diphosphoglycerate and adenosine triphosphate in the erythrocytes was accompanied by an increase in the affinity of the red cells for oxygen, causing reduced oxygen tension in the cells of the body tissues. Zinc is important because of its presence in several vital enzyme systems. Deficiency can result in anemia, splenomegaly, growth failure, and hypogonadism (see Chapter 10). There are also reports that zinc may be important in wound healing and that tissue repair makes substantial demands on the body's zinc reserves. This is particularly important to remember because intravenous nutrition may be necessary in many situations in which these factors are present. Recent studies have demonstrated that chromium is important in maintaining blood sugar levels and that its absence will result in a diabeteslike syndrome. The optimal amount for intravenous nutrition has not been determined yet. Table 5 lists the mineral requirements for adults and infants.

Infusion Techniques

When total parenteral nutrition was first used the central venous catheter had to be introduced with great care and a common complication, which often necessitated removal of the catheter, was infection. Other complications, such as thrombosis and embolism, were also reported. Although these complications still may occur, they are much less frequent today. When short-term intravenous nutrition is required and fat emulsions are being used, a cannula can be inserted into a peripheral vein. It is important not to leave the cannula in the same vein for more than 8 to 12 hours. Complications such as thrombophlebitis do occur but are quite rare. At present central catheters have been inserted in patients and have remained in situ for months and even years without needing to be replaced. Patients have been taught to care for the catheter and to mix and administer their own solutions.

There are several methods for actually administering the solutions. The fat emulsion is usually given separately but can be given through a Y tube.

Table 5.   Mineral requirements

Mineral	Adult (amt/kg/day)	Neonate and Infant (amt/kg/day)
Sodium	1–1.4 mmol	1–2.5 mmol
Potassium	0.7–0.9 mmol	2 mmol
Calcium	0.11	0.5–1 mmol
Magnesium	0.04 mmol	0.15 mmol
Iron	1 μmol	2 μmol
Manganese	0.6 μmol	1 μmol
Zinc	0.3 μmol	0.6 μmol
Copper	0.7 μmol	0.3 μmol
Chlorine	1.3–1.9 mmol	1.8–4.3 mmol
Phosphorus	0.15 mmol	0.4–0.8 mmol
Fluorine	0.7 μmol	3 μmol
Iodine	0.015 μmol	0.04 μmol

The intravenous amino acids are usually given together with the intravenous glucose.

Indications for Total Parenteral Nutrition

In general total parenteral nutrition is employed only when feedings that utilize the gastrointestinal tract are not possible. This situation can be due to the absence or improper functioning of large segments of the GI tract or the inability of the patient to retain anything placed in the GI tract. Partial nutrition, administered by the parenteral route, can be used when the patient is unable to take all of the required nutrients by mouth. Table 6 lists some of the more common indications for intravenous nutrition in adults.

In patients with diseases of the gastrointestinal tract, such as regional enteritis or severe malabsorption, it is occasionally not possible to use oral techniques of any type without exacerbating the disease. Completely resting the bowel for a prolonged period of time either with or without specific therapy may allow enough healing to take place so that oral feedings can be resumed. In patients with GI fistulae this can be extremely important because healing may be accelerated if the bowel is kept empty. In addition such patients often lose significant amounts of fluid through the fistula which must be replaced. Patients with the short bowel syndrome lack

Table 6. Common indications for intravenous nutrition

Gastrointestinal disease
  Chronic inflammatory disease (regional enteritis)
  Short bowel syndrome (infarction or resection)
  Bowel fistulae
    Severe ulcerative colitis
Cancer
  Cachexia due to anorexia
  Preparatory to surgery, chemotherapy, or radiation
Renal failure
    As a method of controlling nitrogen intake (used only when oral therapy is not
  possible)
Hepatic failure
  (Again when oral feeding is not possible)
Surgery and trauma

---

adequate absorptive area, and in cases where the primary cause cannot be repaired long-term or even permanent parenteral nutrition must be used. This is the major indication for the home management programs currently being introduced.

Patients with various types of cancer may become cachetic and emaciated and as a result may not be able to tolerate specific therapy. The major use of parenteral nutrition under these circumstances is as an adjunct to surgery, radiation, or chemotherapy. Studies have shown that patients can be kept in good nutritional status using parenteral nutrition and thereby rendered able to tolerate higher doses of radiation or chemotherapy or better able to withstand a major surgical procedure. Many of the chemotherapeutic agents as well as radiation produce profound nausea and vomiting. Parenteral nutrition is useful in maintaining the patient during this period. Finally, patients are being maintained at home in reasonable comfort on long-term parenteral nutrition, reducing both cost and inconvenience to the patient and his family.

Some patients with chronic renal failure and uremia are unable to take anything by mouth because of nausea and vomiting. Under these conditions dialysis is usually indicated. If for some reason dialysis cannot be done immediately, the patient can be maintained on intravenous nutrition, supplying the essential amino acids and only minimal quantities of the nonessential amino acids. After the BUN has improved, parenteral nutrition can be used together with oral feedings, since many of these patients are unable to consume enough by mouth to maintain good nutritional status.

In acute renal failure, again if the patient cannot consume the diet by mouth, parenteral nutrition with a mixture that supplies nitrogen in limited amounts and mostly as essential amino acids may allow the patient to recover without the use of renal dialysis. In treating patients with severe liver disease, usually in hepatic coma, special solutions must be used. The quantity of aromatic amino acids, such as phenylalanine, tyrosine, and tryptophan must be reduced. Hence the usual solutions cannot be used and special solutions must be mixed. In addition there are some theoretical reasons for using fructose rather than glucose as the major carbohydrate.

In patients who are severely debilitated because of chronic disease or prolonged malnutrition, or both, or in those who cannot eat for prolonged periods of time because of severe trauma, sepsis, or surgical complications, total parenteral nutrition should be carefully planned and undertaken. Such patients invariably lose weight, muscle mass, and total body protein. Parenteral nutrition can significantly reduce nitrogen loss during the height of the catabolic response. In addition it can shorten the period of nitrogen loss and accelerate the recovery process.

Use of Total Parenteral Nutrition in Infants

The same general principles obtain to infants and children as to adults. However, in young infants the indications may be different, the margin of safety is much less, and the complications may be more numerous and severe. Total parenteral nutrition in young infants is indicated in gastrointestinal disease when oral or tube feeding is impossible. This occurs when congenital malformation of the GI tract are present which necessitate neonatal surgery. Examples of these conditions include duodenal and ileal atreasia, malrotation of the bowel, congenital volvulus, and tracheoesophageal fistula. Any major surgery for congenital defects may also necessitate prolonged intravenous feedings.

Certain infants develop chronic and intractable diarrhea from a variety of causes. In the past either oral feedings were continued, often aggravating the diarrhea, in order to keep nutrition adequate, or the patient was given solutions of electrolytes and sugar by vein to rest the GI tract. The latter technique often led to malnutrition and emaciation. With the advent of total parenteral nutrition, a much better method for treating these children has become available. It is now possible to correct electrolyte abnormalities, rest the GI tract, and improve nutritional status simultaneously.

A third group of pediatric patients in whom total parenteral nutrition has been very useful is the very low birth weight infant. It is often very difficult to establish completely adequate enteral intake in very small prematures or small for dates infants. In addition there is concern that malnutrition at this stage of development may affect brain growth and function. The use of intravenous alimentation has prevented the initial weight loss that is seen when enteral feedings alone are employed. Although extensive experience has not yet accumulated in this type of patient, initial results suggest that for selected patients intravenous nutrition can be an important part of therapy.

In feeding any infant parenterally certain precautions must be taken over and above those observed in adults. First, the solutions must contain those amino acids necessary for infants. Second, calories must be of a higher level, usually about 100 to 120/cal/kg of body weight. Third, meticulous attention must be paid to the vitamin and mineral content of the fluid, since margins of safety are much smaller and vitamin deficiency may be more severe. Finally, lipid should be used since essential fatty acid deficiency is more severe in infants and may include the deposition of abnormal myelin (see Chapter 7). Tables 4 and 5 outline the general requirements for young infants. The most common solutions in this country and in Sweden usually meet these requirements. However, some solutions that are used for adults in other countries are not suitable for infants.

Complications

Besides the complications associated with the infusion, infection, thrombophlebitis, and embolism, certain metabolic complications may occur in patients being maintained on total parenteral nutrition. Table 7 outlines these complications.

Most of the metabolic complications associated with total parenteral nutrition can be corrected, if detected early, by altering the composition of the infusate. Therefore it is imperative that any patient on parenteral nutrition be carefully monitored. Acidosis is more common when crystalline amino acid mixtures are used than when protein hydrolysate is used, probably because the arginine and lysine in the hydrochloride salt generate hydrochloric acid regardless of whether they are catabolized or anabolized. If this danger is recognized, it is easily prevented by adding metabolizable base to the infusate. The acidosis could be prevented if the solutions were changed so that arginine and lysine were present as metabolizable salts.

Summary

Total parenteral nutrition is the newest form of alimenting patients unable to retain or assimilate food through the gastrointestinal tract. It is

Table 7.   Metabolic complications of total parenteral nutrition

System Affected	Systemic Disorder
Glucose	Hyperglycemia osmotic diuresis, hyperosmolarity hypoglycemia
Electrolytes	Hyper- or hypo- natremia, kalemia-chloremia
Minerals	Hyper- or hypo- calcemia, phosphatemia, magnesemia
Acid-base	Hyperchloremic metabolic acidosis
Nitrogen Metabolism	Azotemia, hyperammonemia, abnormal plasma aminograms
Vitamins	Hyper- or hypovitaminosis
Fatty acids	Essential fatty acid deficiency
Trace minerals	Zn, Cu deficiencies
Hepatic	Elevated S G O T, S G P T, hepatomegaly

currently used in patients with a variety of illnesses and has significantly improved mortality and morbidity in a number of serious diseases. These include surgery, trauma, burns, GI disease, renal disease, hepatic disease, and various conditions in infancy. Although sufficient calories and nitrogen can be delivered through a central catheter without the use of intravenous lipids, the use of the lipids provides energy in a more physiologic manner and allows the use of peripheral veins. In addition, essential fatty acid deficiency is avoided. The amino acid composition of the fluids is now generally worked out but improvements are still being made. The use of parenteral nutrition is not without risk. Certain complications related to the catheter as well as to the solutions may occur. With the proper team, however, and under the proper circumstances, this new procedure provides new hope for many patients previously condemned to death or to chronic invalidism.

RECOMMENDED READING

Davidson, S., R. Passmore, J. F. Brock, and A. S. Truswell, *Human Nutrition and Dietetics,* Churchill Livingstone, Edinburgh, 1975, pp. 535–545.

Dudrick, S. J., and J. E. Rhoads, New Horizon for Intravenous Feeding, *JAMA,* **215,** 939 (1971).

Fischer, J. E., Ed., *Total Parenteral Nutrition,* Little, Brown, Boston, 1976.

Heird, W. C., and R. Winters, Parenteral Nutrition: Pediatrics, in H. A. Schneider, C. A. Anderson, and D. B. Coursin, Eds., *Nutritional Support of Medical Practice,* Harper and Row, Hagerstown, Md., 1977.

Meng, H. C., Parenteral Nutrition: Principles, Nutrient Requirements, Techniques, and Clinical Applications, in H. A. Schneider, C. E. Anderson, and D. B. Coursin, Eds., *Nutritional Support of Medical Practice,* Harper and Row, Hagerstown, Md., 1977, pp. 152–183.

INDEX